SHEILA KELLEY

THE S FACTOR

STRIP WORKOUTS for EVERY WOMAN

PHOTOGRAPHS BY SHAWN FREDERICK

WORKMAN PUBLISHING • NEW YORK

Library of Congress Cataloging-in-Publication Data
Kelley, Sheila
The S Factor : strip workouts for every woman/by Sheila Kelley.
p. cm.
ISBN 0-7611-3063-2 (alk. paper)—ISBN 0-7611-3257-0 (hc)
1. Exercise for women. 2. Physical fitness for women.
I. Title
GV482.K45 2003
613.7'045--dc21   2003057174

Cover photograph: Davis Factor
Illustrations: Mary Ellen Kelley

Workman books are available at special discounts when purchased in bulk for premiums
and sales promotions as well as for fund-raising or educational use. Special editions or book excerpts
can also be created to specification. For details, contact the Special Sales Director at the address below.

Workman Publishing Company, Inc.
708 Broadway
New York, NY 10003-9555
www.workman.com

Printed in the United States of America

First printing January 2004
10 9 8 7 6 5 4 3 2 1

I dedicate this book to my family—
Richard, Ruby, and Gus,
who make all things in life lush.

And to the original women in my life—
Mom (the hero);
my sisters:
Christine (missing you),
Kitty Kat (the miracle child),
Mary Ellen (Mamie, my twin),
Joyce and Michele (the two other little girls).
You've made my life rich with women.

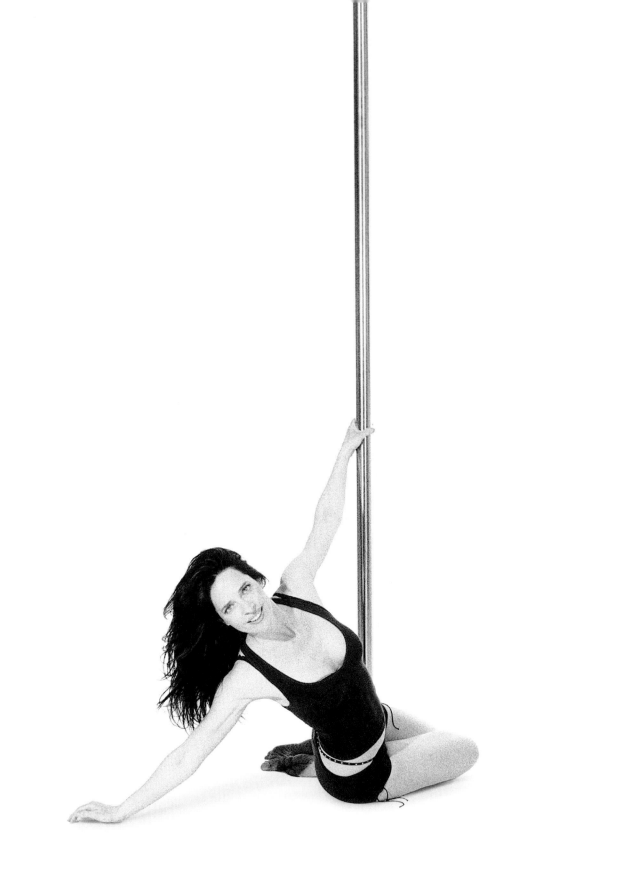

Acknowledgements

I would like to thank the following: all the guys in the family (Dad, Lenny, Gerry, and Patrick), for their love and support; Ruth Sullivan, for her endless efforts and uncompromising vision; Paul Hanson, for his eyes and aesthetic sensibilities; Eve Epstein (my better half), for her inspiration and insight; Sara Goodman and Carrie Brown, for the talks; Merry Lee Traum and Donna Pappas, for their loyalty and love; Cindye Friedman, for her tireless efforts trying to keep up with me; Ilene Feldman, Wendy Murphy, and the whole IFA office, for their belief in me (love you guys!); Shawn Frederick, for the beautiful photos; all my house girls: Sara, Donna, Carrie, Boni, Sally Ann, Kelly, Teri, Gabrielle, Kari, Adria, Julie, Tammara, Karen, Lauren, Vanna, Kathleen P., Nicole, Patty P., Sandy Skinner, Susan Shannon, Corinne, Kathleen C., Megan, Merry Lee, Ruth, Bess, Claire, Alex, Dara, Katelyn, Linda, Stacey Rae, Peri Ellen—you guys blow me away; Juana, Corina, Isolina, and Roxana, for your love and caring; the entire Kelley and Schiff clans, for putting up with my disappearance into the S Factor world; Carolan and Peter Workman, for having the nerve and the belief; Bob DiForio and company, for your persistence; Daphne Ortiz and David Lust, for shining the spotlight; David Linter—for always; Jeanne Heaton, for leading me down the road in the first place; Bill Forsythe, John Sayles, John Boorman, Ridley Scott, and most especially, Michael Hoffman, for seeing; my friends: Michael, Ellie, Rob, Lucinda, John-Jack, Francesca, Bridget, Angela, Earl, and Bob, among others, who keep me sane and happy; the Blue Iguana crew: Devon, Symone, Castle, Nicki, Jezebel, Mili, Millenium, Synne, Daryl, Sandy, Jennifer, Charlotte, Bob, Earl, Elias, Etchie Stroh, Ram Bergman, and Dana Leustig; and Gillette, for the Mach 3, the ultimate in shaving luxury.

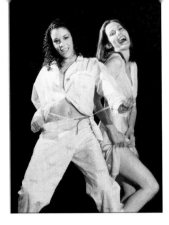

contents

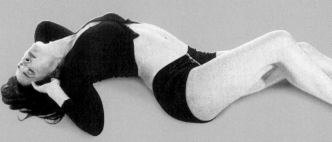

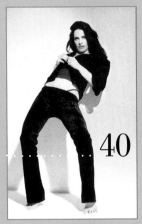

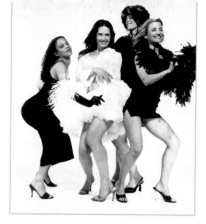

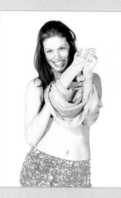
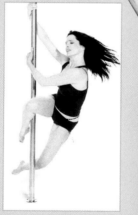
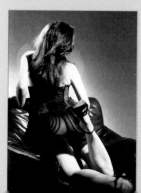

PHOTO BY DAVIS FACTOR

introduction: the origin

O kay, let's get one thing straight. I'm an ordinary, everyday kind of woman. I'm a mother of two with a demanding work schedule and an even more demanding home life. On any given day, I can be seen driving car pool, making marshmallow squares for the PTA, or zooming frantically from a film shoot to teaching to an audition—usually dressed in a scruffy T-shirt and

of the s factor

a pair of jeans. If I'm lucky, I sneak in a shower before 9:00 P.M. In other words, I'm probably a lot like you.

Except for one thing. I have a stripper's pole in my husband's office.

I love to pole-dance and strip; I do it every day of the week (except Sundays—even the obsessed need a break). I don't do it for money, and I don't do it for strangers. I stripdance for myself, and—if he's been very, very good—I strip for my husband. I do it because it makes me look and feel extraordinary. Because it lets me soar high above the world and its troubles. Because when I dance, layers of self-doubt and self-consciousness fall away to reveal my true, powerful self. I do it, in short, because it has

changed my life and continues to change it.

Let me tell you the story of how a seemingly normal person like me discovered a secret in the unlikeliest corner of the world—a secret that has helped hundreds of women face down their greatest fears and achieve their greatest aspirations. It's the story of the S Factor, a movement technique based on the athleticism and sexual expression of stripping and pole dancing, derived from the natural S-like curvature of the female body. It's my story, but it's also the beginning of yours: the first step on a journey that will take you to parts of yourself you may have lost touch with or perhaps never knew existed.

As the title suggests, this book will teach you how to move like a stripper, how to give a great lap dance, and how to perform pole tricks. It will provide you with a new workout routine that will reshape your body. It will add a healthy dose of excitement to your love life. But it will do more than that. For me and the women I teach, the S Factor is the best way we've found to gain confidence, self-knowledge, and physical awareness—all while having a ridiculously good time.

The Beginning

My fascination with stripping began fourteen years ago, when I was a young, hungry actress researching one of my first paying roles. I had been cast as a prostitute and stripper named Carrie in the film *Breaking In,* and in the interest of research I decided to visit a strip club. I didn't relish the thought: I'd been raised a nice Irish Catholic girl, and I considered myself a staunch feminist. I believed strip clubs to be the province of the desperate and the depraved.

So I was skeptical and a little scared as I pulled up outside Star Strip, a club on the outskirts of Beverly Hills. It was 2:00 P.M. on a Wednesday, and despite the darkness of the club, I could see that the place was nearly empty. I grabbed a seat in the back,

hunched my shoulders, and pulled my collar up around my neck. It took a while before I found the courage to look up at the stage.

A young, blond, shaggy-haired dancer stood—no, towered—above a middle-aged man sitting below her. She was almost completely naked, and in the yellow gleam of the stage lights her flesh gave off a hot glow, as if lit from within. The slow, undulating movements of her hips had a mesmerizing effect that seemed to emanate from somewhere deep inside her, a place of power and knowledge that transcended the sleaziness of her surroundings. Her gaze was fierce, triumphant. In that moment, she looked nothing like the victimized, objectified creature I'd expected to see. And there was something about the rapt expression of the man at her feet that made the moment even more intense. She was, in that moment, a goddess worthy of worship and adulation.

Then the song ended, the man threw two bucks at her, the spell was broken, and the power faded from her eyes.

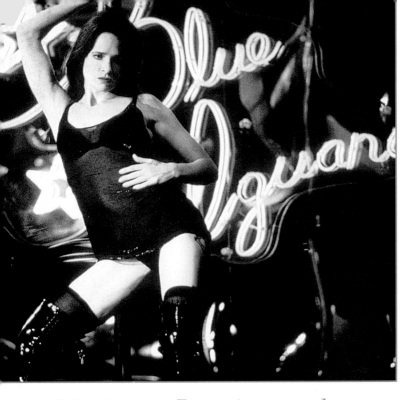

Sheila as Stormy in Dancing at the Blue Iguana.

Dancing at the Blue Iguana

That moment stayed with me. I knew I had witnessed something extraordinary. Yes, strip clubs were unsavory places where exploitation was the norm. But there was something else going on there, and it fascinated me. The movement was so unbelievably beautiful, it didn't seem to belong in such a shady and decadent place.

I started to write a script about a young stripper in Hollywood. Several years and even more rewrites later, this script became *Dancing at the Blue Iguana,* an improvisational film set in the San Fernando Valley. As an actress in the film whose job it was to create a character and story line,

I realized that it was time to return to the clubs, this time to be more than an observer.

Crazy Girls, a club in the heart of Los Angeles, became my classroom. Two strippers in particular, Symone and Devon, became my teachers. Both were extraordinary dancers, amazing athletes, and true artists. Symone, a dark and captivating loner, moved with long, sharp glides and quick turns. She could levitate her body out to the side of the pole like a Cirque du Soleil performer. Devon was sensuality personified, like Jessica Rabbit on opium, moving her body dreamily from one slow body undulation to the next.

As I watched and worked with them, I began to realize that stripping and pole work were not techniques that had ever been "taught"; the moves these women knew so well had been passed on through an unspoken osmosis, a watch-and-learn system. In other words, these chicks were great dancers but not the greatest instructors. If I wanted to learn, I'd have to study, analyze, and break down the movement myself.

And that's what I did. Over the next several months, I not only mastered the basic moves of stripping and pole dancing, but I also found that as I made these moves my own, my film character's persona emerged. She was dark, powerful, and mysterious, a force of nature, an explosive tempest with a tranquil stillness at its core. I named her Stormy.

After a few weeks of practicing, I began to notice amazing changes in my body. I was thirty-four years old, but I was beginning to look the way I had when I was twenty-four. Dancing every day had melted away my postpregnancy fat (my son was four) and defined the muscles in my arms, legs, and stomach. The lower back pain I'd had for years from a high-school injury disappeared. I dropped an entire jean size, and felt energetic and alive. For the first time in my life, I became confident in my body and stopped judging myself. When I looked in the mirror, I no longer saw the flaws, the wrinkles, and the cellulite. Instead, I saw a lithe, sensual creature. A woman who knew her own strength.

As I grew more confident, I started performing at L.A. clubs during the day before the crowds descended. Two weeks before filming, I danced at a few places at night. Then I gave myself the ultimate test: I invited my husband, Richard, to come as a patron.

It was at a club called Spice Lady. Nobody there knew I was an actress preparing for a role. And, man, was I a nervous wreck. I've performed to live audiences as large as 1,400 and as small as twelve, but never in my life have I felt as terrified as I did that night when I handed my music to the DJ. My breath was short, my hands

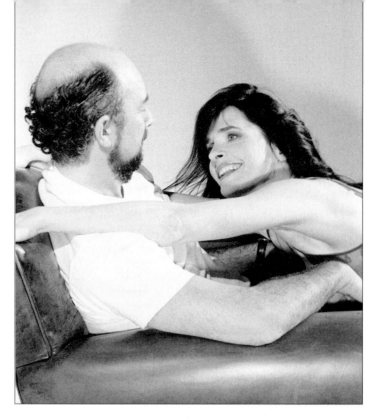

were sweaty (which is catastrophic for pole work), and my heart was pounding. Richard walked through the door and took a seat in front of the stage. Our eyes met and we smiled. And then the DJ called for Stormy.

As Led Zeppelin's "When the Levy Breaks" started, I took one last breath and let the heavy drumbeat pick me up like a wave, and before I knew it, I was up and down the pole, twirling, suspended, aloft. My body took over and, with an innate physical wisdom I'd never experienced before, moved with total freedom and integrity. I crawled over to Richard like a lioness stalking her prey, stopped in front of him and slowly circled my hips. Richard sat transfixed. He gazed at me, breathed me

Richard Schiff and Sheila Kelly: A perfect moment in a beautiful marriage.

in, his face full of awe. As we locked into each other's eyes, we transcended the seediness of the club. It was a perfect moment—a moment that went on and on, and one that has become a milestone in a beautiful and remarkable marriage. Richard then hired me to do a lap dance. And may I say he got the best damn lap dance of his life.

And then I did what no stripper should do: I went home with my "customer."

Sheila pole dances alone—flying untethered and free.

My Own Perfect Moment

Nine months later, and after we finished filming *Dancing at the Blue Iguana*, I gave birth to a baby girl. (I told you it was the best lap dance ever.) And for a while, my sexual identity disappeared inside a big Mother Earth goddess. I was carrying around extra fat from nursing, and I felt like a fleshy, sluggish milk cow, totally disconnected from my sexual self. Motherhood was wonderful, but I started thinking about how great I'd felt when I'd been stripping—how solid and strong my body had been, how much energy and vitality had coursed through my veins. I wanted that body back. I wanted that feeling back.

One day, I started fantasizing about putting a pole up in Richard's office out back. At first I tried to talk myself out of it. "Sheila, that was a role. This is real life. You're a wife and mother, for God's sake." But it was no use. Somewhere inside, I had already made up my mind.

I installed the pole the next day.

Dancing felt different this time. I started dancing an hour a day, and after several weeks of hard work, bruised knees, and pole burns, I felt my body and sexuality returning. It was making me more confident, more self-knowing, and more fulfilled. But this time I wasn't doing it for Richard. I wasn't doing it for a role. I was doing it for myself.

One afternoon in March, I had an experience that brought this revelation home. I had put on one of my favorite Clash songs. I began moving, and in that instant something switched on in me. I was moving without a moment's forethought or self-consciousness; my body became like a river of sinew and muscle and raw energy. There was no one there but me. Leaning back against the wall with my hips jutting out unapologetically, I slid languorously to the floor like slow molasses. Once on the floor, I allowed the music to curve and shape me with its wave. Then I was up, swinging around the pole, flying, untethered and free. I moved with complete physical and sensual intuition, and for the first time, totally for myself. There was no audience, no camera crew, no man. My body felt solid and strong, yet at the same time fluid, lithe, molten. I felt like a bad ass and an angel all at once. This wasn't the same high I'd had the night I danced for Richard. It was sharper, fiercer, more vivid. This was about me. I felt luminous.

The S Factor Is Born

I started joking with my friends that I was going to teach them how to strip. "Forget yoga. Forget weight training. Forget therapy," I said. "Stripping brings you inner peace, erotic power, and a great body." They thought I was kidding. I wasn't.

I gave my first class on April 18, 2001, to just four students: a businesswoman, a screenwriter, a personal trainer, and a nutritionist. Having analyzed and broken down the movements into steps during my own learning process, I found that teaching it came easily. I refined the class into a

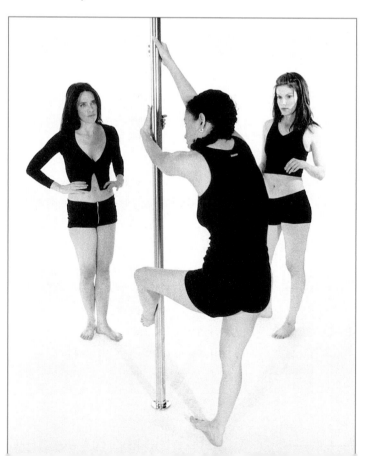

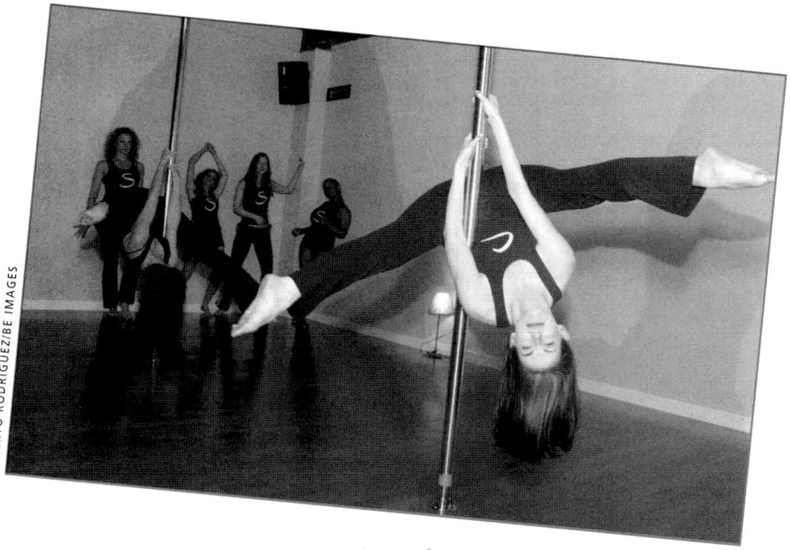
ALBERTO RODRIGUEZ/BE IMAGES

workout that went beyond stripping and pole tricks (though they remain key elements in the S Factor workout) and distilled the principles of natural, circular, female movement into a unique system that empowers and strengthens the whole woman, inside and out. I dubbed it the S Factor, after the innate female S shape that forms the basis for the movements and the technique.

Left and above: a beginner and an advanced class in the S Factor studio in Los Angeles.

In just six classes, I saw my students transformed. Faces that had been set and tense became soft and relaxed. Women who walked into class with the baggage of life on their shoulders walked out as though they could conquer the world. Over time, their bodies became firmer and leaner. I heard about improvements in their relationships with their lovers, husbands, and friends. I witnessed students celebrating their bodies and their classmates' bodies. They stopped judging themselves, and they stopped judging other women.

My classes grew and grew. Today I teach more than a hundred women each week. In June of 2003, I opened a new S Factor studio in Los Angeles and have trained six teachers, who also have full schedules. I get e-mails from women all over the world who want to learn how to strip and pole dance. I realized that I wanted to spread the word even further, and decided to write a book that gave women the techniques (and the permission!) to do what I had done. In your hands is the key and an invitation to join the growing community of women who have discovered the secret of sensual movement and erotic dance.

My students are a lot like you. They are young and old, from myriad backgrounds, and their bodies come in all shapes and sizes. They are maverick explorers, brave women entering uncharted territory within themselves and the world. They are my heroes. And they remind me every day of why I do what I do. I invite you to join their ranks.

chapter one: *meet your*

There exists in every woman a hidden erotic creature, a center of sexual power and self-knowledge. She may be buried beneath a pinstriped business suit or lie next to a man whose snores lull her to sleep; she may hide in a body whose owner lives in mortal fear of full-length mirrors and bikinis. But trust me: she's there. She's the wild, feline, untamed part of you, your sexual

erotic creature

alter ego—and the opposite of the "good girl" or "little lady." Some of us know her better than others do, but I would venture to guess that your erotic creature hasn't seen nearly enough light of day.

By nature, women are sensual beings. Our breasts protrude, our butts stick out, our hips curve, and our waists indent. Many of us have been conditioned to hide or diminish this sensuality; we've been told to keep our hips straight, our butts tucked, and our breasts well hidden. Even most exercise programs (aerobics, step, spinning, weight lifting) and some dance practices (ballet, tap) teach us to square the hips and keep the body linear and rigid. The S Factor challenges this "male" paradigm of square, angular movement. It teaches you to move your body in circular, sinuous motions and to exaggerate those movements so that you make yourself bigger and fill space with your shapes and your curves. It will allow your body to move in more fluid and supple ways.

The S Factor movements themselves will begin to put you in touch with your sensual self. But

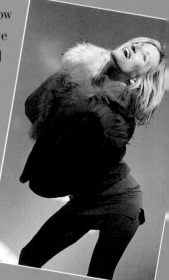

getting to know your inner erotic creature will take some time and energy. Who is she? She's different for every woman. For you she might be a playful 1940s pinup, a Montana Cowgirl, a pretty-in-pink Baby Doll, a black-leather-clad Rocker Chick, a bespectacled Marian the Librarian, a French maid, or an elegant Park Avenue seductress. At times, she may be a combination of many different things. Your erotic creature has moods that evolve over time and defy simple labels. In other words, she's as idiosyncratic as you are.

Consider this book a guide to discovering your erotic self and bringing her out of hiding. The exercises at the end of each chapter should help. I encourage you to record moments in your journal when you catch a glimpse of her. Is there a song, smell, place, person, or even time of day that seems to draw her out more? The longer you practice the S Factor, the more evidence you'll collect about this sensual self and the more fully she'll emerge.

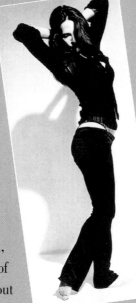

Useful Terms

The following are terms and directions that will be used repeatedly throughout the exercises in this book. It's important that you become familiar with them now.

Sit bones: The ischial tuberosities or, to put it in common language, the large, nerveless bones at the base of your pelvic girdle that you sit upon.

Scoop your belly: A term used in Pilates that means to suck your abdominal muscles in as though you were trying to touch your belly button to your spine.

Arch your back: Push the middle of your spine as far forward as you can, keeping your shoulders back and pushing your chest forward.

Lengthen your foot: Point the entire foot, extending the line of the leg from the hip all the way through the toes. (Do not simply point the toes; point the entire foot.)

Peel: Moving one thing away from another—feeling that bit of resistance that holds them together.

WARMING UP

The S Factor begins with slow, circular warm-up movements that serve a dual purpose: they prepare your body for the more rigorous exercises to come and they give you a feel for the grace and fluidity that your body will ultimately achieve. First, make sure you have the following:

A space. Choose a place that feels safe and private. It should have at least one free wall and enough floor space for you to be able to make a "snow angel." (If you're working out with a group, make sure everyone can do snow angels simultaneously without creating an unintentional kickboxing scene.)

A mat. It can be a basic yoga mat, but I recommend something thicker—I use ¼-inch mats because they cushion the knees and head.

A mirror. Full-length is fine, but a dressing-room mirror is even better. If you're working out alone, your mirror is your teacher: it will help you see and then correct and adjust your body to follow along with the photos and illustrations in this book.

Workout clothes. Wear something comfortable that you can move easily in. You can jump right in with something that feels sexy, but most of my students come to their first few classes in sweatpants and tank tops. There's plenty of time to explore sexier, more playful clothing once you've gotten more confident with the movements.

A journal. Use a journal to give voice to the emotions that arise as you work through the movements, as well as for the writing assignments at the end of the chapters. In the absence of feedback from a class and teacher, a journal will allow you to express yourself and then to look back and chart your progress. Think of it as a stand-in for me. Confide in your journal, let it become a sounding board and a playground for your mind, just as the S Factor is a playground for your body.

Music. Have a cassette or CD player with at least an hour's worth of music that you love and that relaxes you. For each type of exercise in the book, I recommend a number of selections I like or have found successful in class.

sitting spine circles

Adapted from Kundalini yoga, this exercise focuses on spinal energy. Feel your sit bones pressing into the mat and imagine that they are rooting you to the ground. Now imagine your head is filled with helium, so that your spine is being pulled up at the same time that it is being pulled down by your sit bones, creating a wonderful and dynamic stretch of the spine.

TIME: 10 seconds per circle

body benefit:
Sitting Spine Circles open the hips and work the core muscles in your abdomen and back. This increases blood flow to the pelvic region and promotes the health of the reproductive organs.

1 Sit in an easy cross-legged position with your left foot in front of your right and your hands resting on your knees.

Increase the size of your spine circles with each inhalation until you're making large circles that stretch your spine in every direction.
Do ten clockwise; change direction and repeat.

6 Inhale as you come around to the front again, pushing your chest out in front of you and arching your back.

2 Inhale and push your chest out toward the wall in front of you like the carved figure on the prow of a ship, arching your back and neck.

3 Begin circling your spine clockwise, pushing your spine around to the right. Be sure to keep your left sit bone on the mat. Feel the stretch in the right side of your torso.

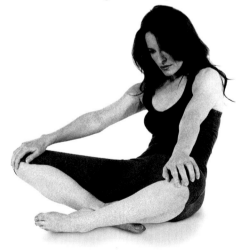

5 Circle the middle of your spine around to the left. Feel the stretch in the left side of your torso. Keep your right sit bone on the mat.

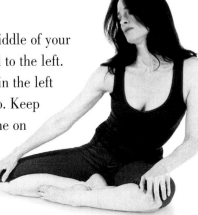

4 As you come around to the back, exhale and push the middle of your spine out toward the wall behind you. Scoop in your belly, creating a large semicircle with your upper body.

inverted spine circles

These circles involve moving your entire upper body while keeping your hips and pelvis still. If your head had a paintbrush sprouting from the top of it, you'd be painting a smooth circle on the floor around you in this exercise.

TIME: 10 seconds per circle

body benefit:
This stretch enhances movement of the spine—the vertebrae, the discs, ligaments, and muscles. One of the reasons many of us experience chronic back pain is because we have limited range of motion in our spines. Unlike muscles that are nourished through blood flow, the discs between your vertebrae receive nourishment through the circulation of synovial fluid—and this circulation occurs only through movement and stretching.

sensual focus:
Focus on the feeling of openness this exercise gives you—opening your ribs, chest, throat, heart, and back to the world. How does the exposure affect you? Does it bring up any emotions? Allow these feelings to come out through the movement, rather than pushing them away.

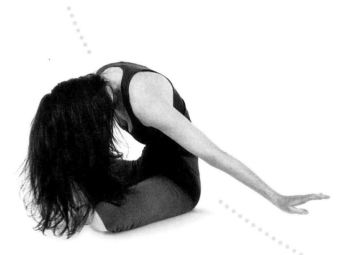

1 Sit in an easy cross-legged position, with your left foot in front of your right and your hands resting on your knees.

Continue circling, exhaling when forward, inhaling when back, ten times. Then change directions and repeat.

6 Exhale as you sweep your head around to the front, scooping your belly and pushing your lower back out toward the wall behind you.

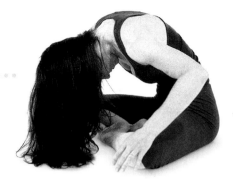

2 Drop your head and upper torso forward. Exhale as you scoop your belly and push your lower back out toward the wall behind you. Imagine you are cradling a beach ball in your lap.

3 Begin to circle your head and shoulders clockwise, bringing them around to the right. Feel the stretch in the left side of your torso. Keep both sit bones on the floor.

4 Circle your head to the back as you inhale, placing your hands flat on the floor behind you for support. Arch your back and open your chest up toward the ceiling.

5 Continue to circle around to the left, feeling the stretch in the right side of your torso. Again, remember to keep both sit bones on the floor.

TRANSITION

to Open Leg Stretches
Roll up your spine vertebra by vertebra until you are sitting tall, with your back and neck straight. Slowly unfold the left leg with the foot lengthened, then unfold the right leg so the two are in a straddling position.

→

open leg stretch

I adapted this stretch from ballet, which I studied for many years. Throughout this continuous movement, keep your pelvis anchored to the floor as though it is embedded in a block of cement.

TIME: 2 minutes per cycle

body benefit:
The Open Leg Stretch gives a comprehensive stretch to the entire back, from the skull to the heels, increasing flexibility in the lumbar spine and hips.

1 Sit in a straddle position, feet lengthened and torso upright.

Drag your left hand along the floor back to the center. Allow your head to follow, then your right hand, until you've **RETURNED TO STEP 2.**
Repeat in opposite direction: begin by dragging the right hand back toward the right ankle.

5 Raise your torso upright and to the center. Extend your left hand above your head; now inhale and stretch your torso to the right with your chest facing the wall in front of you, your right shoulder pointing toward your right knee, and your right hand on your right ankle. Exhale and turn your chest in toward the right knee.

2 Exhale as you walk your hands forward between your knees, keeping your lower back straight, reaching your lower abdomen toward the floor as far as you can go. Inhale deeply, imagining that you are drawing breath directly into the muscles of your lower back and pelvis. Exhale.

Inhale and flex your feet. Exhale and point your feet.

3 Slowly sweep your left hand over to your left ankle, then your head, followed by your right hand. Keeping your back flat, exhale and lower your chest toward the left knee. Keep your right hip firmly planted on the floor and your feet lengthened.

4 Rotate your torso so that your chest is facing the wall in front of you. Stretch your left shoulder toward your left knee. Extend your right arm above your head. Lengthen your spine, imagining that your upper torso is diving out of your pelvis.

LUXURY OF MOVEMENT

Even though some of them are strenuous, all of the movements in this workout should feel natural and sensual. That's the goal here: true sensuality, the ability to dwell in the luxury of each muscular movement and take as much pleasure in it as possible. Getting to that point takes some time and requires retraining your brain as well as your body. Below are some reminders to get you into an S Factor mind-set.

Slow down. Nothing is more powerful or more erotic than a woman who takes her time. Find your internal metronome and follow it. Use your breath to help you.

There are physical benefits to slowing down, too. When you move quickly, gravity and momentum take the burden off your muscles. When you move slowly, your muscles must initiate and sustain each movement, which gives the body a much more thorough workout.

Feel the stretch. Find the deepest, fullest stretch in each position and movement: the roundest arch of your neck, the farthest twist of your spine, the longest forward stretch of your leg as you take a step.

Use deliberate movements. Move your body through the exercises with clear intent and self-assurance. Think economy of motion: use the least amount of movement in the longest amount of time. Pay attention not so much to where you are going as to how you're getting there. And try to stay in the moment.

Visualize. As you move, imagine that you're pushing your body through a thick, viscous substance like molasses or hot fudge. Feel the resistance in such places as your chest and back, your hips and legs and arms.

Use all five senses. Pay attention to the sensations of a single, isolated part of your body. For example, observe the feel of your hair on your shoulders and face when you roll your head back; feel the tops of your feet on the carpet or mat as you kneel and circle your hips. Notice how the light in the room plays across your body and face. Become aware of the taste in your mouth, the smell of your skin, your hair, your clothes. Feel the waves of sound surrounding your body. In many of the exercises, I suggest a specific sensual focus to get you started. But in the future, feel free to come up with some of your own.

BREATH

Every movement in the workout should be propelled by an inhalation or an exhalation. Your breath should fuel the motion of your body like wind in a sail. For example, in the Sitting Spine Circles, note how the inhalation pushes your chest forward, out and open, while the exhalation draws your belly back into a scooped position. Likewise, as your chest comes out, it pulls the breath in.

Deep breathing is essential to every exercise in the book; it increases your body's ability to stretch by delivering more oxygen to your cells. Try this experiment: During the Open Leg Stretch, with your torso bent between your legs, *inhale* (but hold your position), drawing fresh oxygen into the muscles in your lower back. Then *exhale* deeply and sink deeper into the stretch. You might be surprised at how the breath allows you to expand or extend farther in whatever exercise you are doing.

reclining
quad stretch

Y ou will be using your quadriceps a great deal throughout the S Factor workout, so you need to warm them up with this required stretch. You may begin by using your elbow or hand for support, but make it a goal to work up to a full stretch with your back on the floor. With the Reclining Quad Stretch, you'll also begin to explore the power of touch. (See page 16.)

TIME: 45 seconds per side

1 Sit with your legs straight out in front of you, keeping your feet lengthened.

6 Roll over onto your right side and push back up into a sitting position. Unfold the bent leg and extend it out next to the outstretched one as in step 1. Repeat on the other side.

5 Breathe deeply as you slowly move your right hand down your left arm and across your chest and breasts. Move it over your belly, your groin, and around to your hips and butt.

2 Rock back on your right sit bone and fold your left leg back so that your foot is resting, sole up, next to your left buttock.

3 Exhale and slowly lower your back toward the floor using your outstretched hands to control your movement backward.

4 Inhale and stretch your arms up over your head. Stretch up and to the left, then up and to the right. Breathe into the stretch and relax your quad muscles.

Beginner Modification

If the stretch is too intense, lean back only onto your hand or elbow. Instead of raising both arms above your head, raise only one of them as you keep the other on the floor.

breaking the taboo of touch

Throughout the S Factor workout, you will be asked to move your hand over your body. It may feel strange at first; many of us are taught to fear our own flesh and to be embarrassed by the sensations that touching produces. But it's less scary than it seems—you're simply getting to know the topography of your body. Don't be afraid of the parts of your body associated with sex. It's your body; you have a right to know it. The purpose of the touching exercises is to get to know your body more intimately than anyone else ever will. To help you focus, take one of the following approaches to touch.

The Explorer

Think of your hands as those of a scientist or an explorer. Focus on . . .

Texture. Observe the varying degrees of roughness of your skin—how much softer the underside of your arm is than your elbow. Notice the change of texture from skin to cloth, cloth to hair.

Shape. Allow your hands to define the shape that your body cuts in space, the amount of room it takes up, its abundance of curves. Try to discover a curve you didn't know you had—your underarm leading into your breast, for example.

The Physical Healer

Hold your hands close to, but not touching, your face. Feel the heat emanating from them? That's healing energy that can bring warmth and strength to any discomfort in your body.

Let your hands be drawn to the physical aches and pains in your body. The bad back, the injured knee, the stomachache, the sore muscles, the headache. Linger on these spots as you feel the warmth of your hands soothe away tension and pain.

The Emotional Soother

Your hands' soothing power can help heal emotional pains as well as physical ones. As your hands ride along the surface of your body, let them trace the emotions inside. Find the spots in your body that are filled with joy and light.

Physical tightness and emotional repression are linked. Where does your body hold sadness? Love? Anger? Jealousy?

Coax your hand to go to the places where you hold sorrow, anxiety, or painful memories, or where you just feel something locked, tight, resisting movement. Let your hands linger there, soothing and drawing out these negative feelings like a magnet.

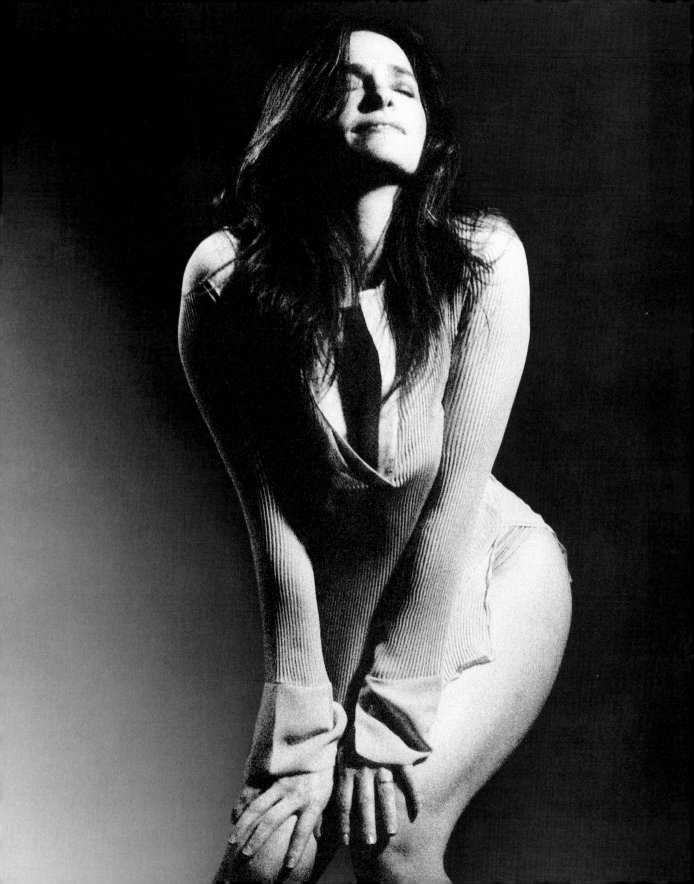

RIPPLE EFFECT

The warm-up portion of this program launches you immediately into an awareness of your sensuality. Go with it. Explore it. For many students, learning this new movement makes them feel downright euphoric; they feel lighter on their feet and have a sense of self-discovery. Others find it hard to get beyond the taboos involved with moving their bodies so freely (and overtly). They still struggle with body issues and societal pressures.

That's why I like using the word "stripping" in the book; it is a metaphor for the journey that takes place in me and my students. We are stripping away layers of social conditioning, negativity, and criticism. The desire to control women's erotic power practically defines our culture. We absorb our culture's negative messages; we experience our sexual selves as threatening, embarrassing, or off-limits. Confide in your journal. It's a safe place to explore the emotions and thoughts that might come up as you unlock your sensuality.

On the facing page are some negative messages that often get replayed in our heads, especially when we think about doing something as seemingly taboo as stripping. Look over the list and check any statements that you relate to.

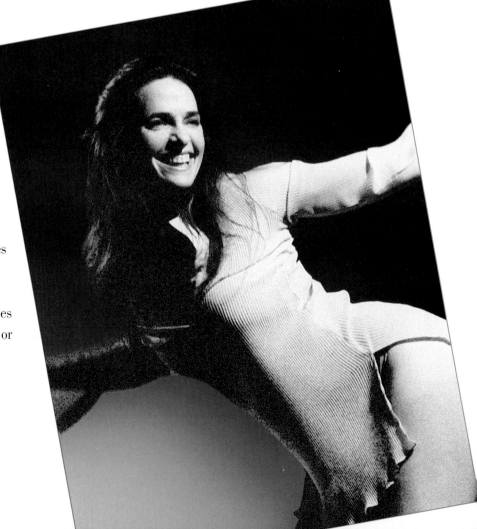

I Can't Strip Because . . .

- ☐ I will look/feel silly.
- ☐ It's dirty.
- ☐ I'm too fat.
- ☐ I'm too old.
- ☐ People will laugh at me.
- ☐ I'm just not naturally sexy.
- ☐ It's a sin.
- ☐ It's not motherly.
- ☐ I will become oversexed.
- ☐ I will be less attractive/coordinated/sexy/thin than other women.
- ☐ I will be tempting men to come on to me.
- ☐ I have no rhythm.
- ☐ I hate my

_____.

(Fill in any body part that may apply.)

Now go through each checked statement and ask yourself: Where did this message come from? Who first said these things to you? Did the idea come from you or from someone else's standards or rules?

In your journal, write about any emotions that come up for you and the origin of these emotions.

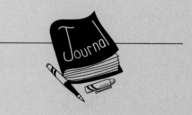

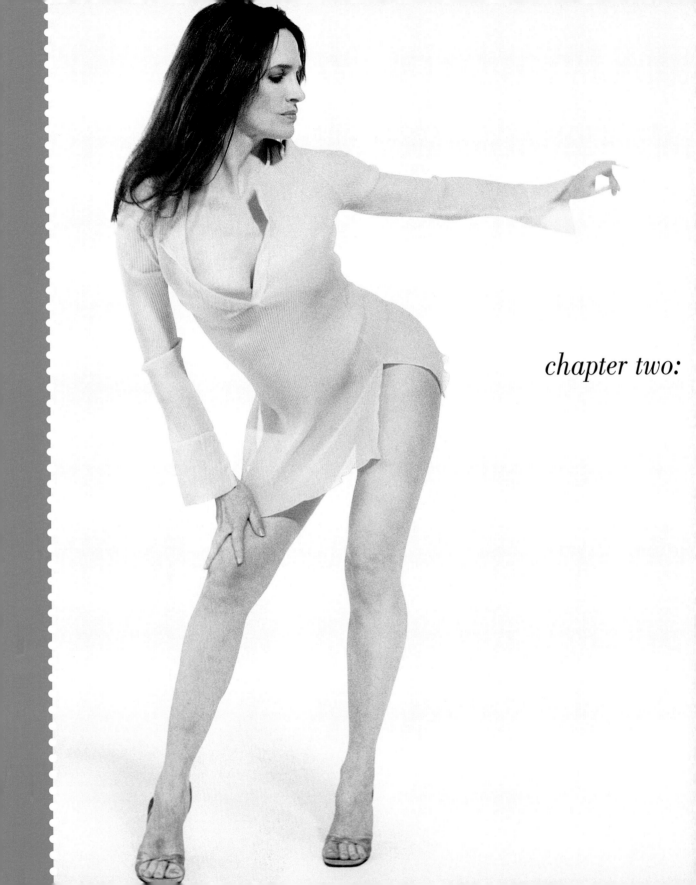

chapter two:

As the Talking Heads so eloquently observed, "The world moves on a woman's hips." One of the first breakthroughs in S Factor movement is to unlock your hips and free them to go where they want to go and do what they want to do. The core movement in the S Factor is the hip circle; many of the exercises are built around it. The movements in this chapter will

hip talk

begin to unlock the power in your pelvis. You'll feel the physical changes in your body almost immediately as you start to push the boundaries of how far you can stretch and move yourself.

You may also unblock some powerful feelings as you release your hips. The reason for this is that we tense certain muscles to keep emotions from coming out. Over time, this tension locks muscles. When you

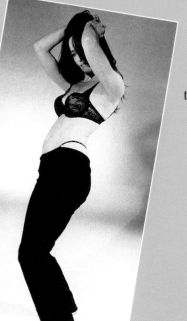

begin to stretch and move your body in ways that it's unaccustomed to, it sometimes triggers the original emotion and you may experience a powerful release. If this happens, take a deep, cleansing breath and continue to move your body through the exercise and through the feelings.

brain massage

Ever notice how good it feels to have your scalp massaged? That's because we hold so much of our tension in our heads. This exercise uses a gentle hip circle to create a wonderful massage of the entire skull in an attempt to turn the brain off and let the body take over. As you do this, try to imitate how a cat looks when it's rolling its head in catnip.

TIME: 5 seconds per circle

body benefit:
The nerve endings in your scalp are the end points for all of your nerves, so you should feel the effects of this massage throughout your entire body. The Brain Massage also releases endorphins.

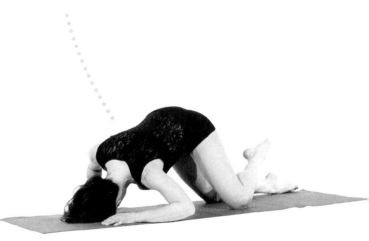

1 Kneel on your hands and knees. Keep your lower back arched, abs tight.

RETURN TO STEP 2, Ruby's pose. Do ten head rolls in each direction.

5 Inhale as you circle your butt back and around to the right, allowing the left side of your skull to roll against the mat.

2 On an inhalation, bring your chest and head down toward the floor until your right cheek is resting on your mat. Your butt is sticking straight up in the air and your hands should be on the mat next to your head. I call this "Ruby's pose," because it looks just like my two-year-old daughter when she's sleeping.

3 Exhale and push your weight forward so that you roll onto the top of your scalp. (Do not rest all your weight on your head; rather, allow just enough of it to apply pressure on your scalp and a gentle stretch to your neck.)

4 As you come forward, tuck in your belly and push your lower back up toward the ceiling. Try to let the top or even back of your skull roll against the mat.

cat-cow wave

This move involves two yoga positions, the Cat and the Cow, which I have modified for the S Factor. Keep the image of a constant, endless wave in your mind as you do this.

TIME: 10 seconds per wave

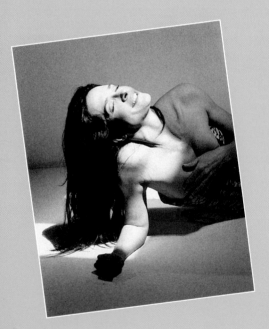

1 Get on your hands and knees, with your hands about shoulder-width apart and your knees a little more than hip-width apart.

Keep the undulation smooth and continual, like a wave on the surface of the ocean. Allow your body's movement to move the air in and out of your body.

Repeat ten times.

4 Starting at the pelvis, exhale as you roll your spine back up again toward the ceiling, dropping your head and scooping your belly into the Cat.

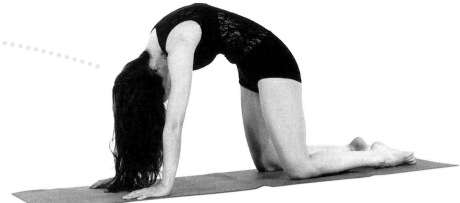

2 **Cat:** Tuck your pelvis and drop your head. Exhale as you roll your back up toward the ceiling as high as it can go, like a Halloween cat.

PLAYLIST **Surge & Urge**

 You can begin to pick up the pace of the music, but its predominant quality should still be flowing and wavelike.

* Coldplay, *Parachutes:* "Yellow," "We Never Change," "Trouble"
* Aerosmith, *Toys in the Attic:* "Sweet Emotion"
* Buddy Guy, *Sweet Tea:* "Baby, Please Don't Leave"
* Lynyrd Skynyrd, *All Time Greatest Hits:* "Simple Man"
* Moby, *Play:* "If Things Were Perfect"

3 **Cow:** Starting with the pelvis, inhale and lower your spine vertebra by vertebra as you lift your head and arch your back until your belly almost touches the mat. Allow your elbows to bend, but not touch the mat. Keep your abdominal muscles tight to support your lower back.

cat-cow roll

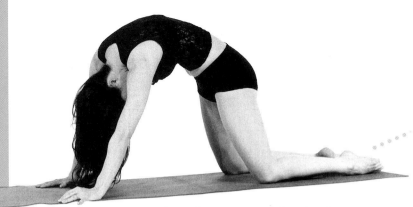

This exercise connects the Cat-Cow Wave with a more circular motion. Focus on making the biggest, most delicious circles with your upper body that you can. As you do this, imagine yourself kneeling inside a barrel or a tube, and try to touch its inside surface all the way around with your upper torso.

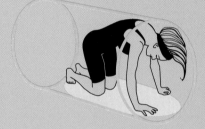

TIME: 10 seconds per roll

1 Continue from the position of the Cat-Cow Wave. Exhale as you roll your spine up toward the ceiling, scoop your belly, and drop your head toward the mat.

Repeat ten times. Then reverse the movement and repeat it ten times to the right.

5 Exhale as you roll your spine up toward the ceiling, with your belly scooped and your head dropped toward the mat.

2 Circle your spine to the left, pushing out to the side with the left side of your torso, feeling the stretch in your rib cage and opening your waist.

3 Sweep your chest and abdomen down toward the floor as you inhale, arching your back. Support your weight with your bent arms; do not rest your chest on the floor.

4 Circle your spine to the right, pushing out to the side with the right side of your torso, feeling the stretch in your rib cage and opening up your waist.

rocking cat

This exercise takes the Cat-Cow undulation to another level, engaging the hips and creating a ripple effect throughout the entire body. You'll be circling your hips in an oval, parallel to the floor. Like the Cat-Cow Roll, it's a stunning, sensual movement that can be incorporated into any routine. It's also a strenuous move, so keep the breath flowing.

Keep your movement fluid and deliberate. Many muscles come into play and you want to make sure not to skip any of them, so take your time. Note how, with the circular movement of the hips, your entire body, including the head and neck, become involved.

TIME: 10 seconds per rotation

body focus:

Arching your back compresses the spine and rejuvenates the spinal nerves by bringing a rich supply of blood to this region, as well as massaging and toning the back muscles. The Rocking Cat movement also brings in a fresh supply of sinovial fluid to the joints, which nourishes the joint cavity and surrounding structures.

1 Kneel on your mat, hands a little more than shoulder-width apart, knees about hip-width apart.

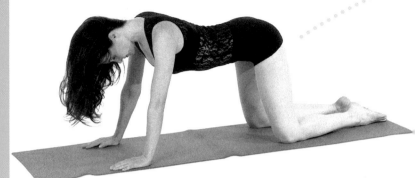

RETURN TO STEP 2 by rotating your hips around to the back, with your arms outstretched. Repeat ten times. Reverse the movement and do ten repetitions in the opposite direction.

5 Rotate your hips and torso around to the right, opening up your rib cage. Imagine you are trying to touch the right wall with your right hip.

2 Arch your back as you inhale, stick your butt straight up, and stretch your arms out in front of you on the floor, head down—like a cat stretching.

3 Rotate your hips and torso to the left, opening up your rib cage. *Playful modification*: Throw a "kick" into it by pointing and lifting the right foot.

4 Exhale and bring your hips forward so that they almost touch the floor. Support yourself by keeping your abdominal muscles fully engaged and your shoulders down. Do not "fall" into the pose.

kneeling
hip circles

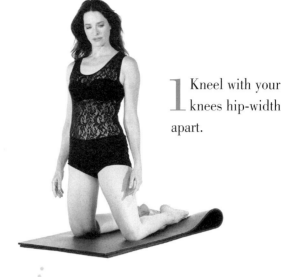

1 Kneel with your knees hip-width apart.

In this move, again, you want to stretch as far as possible in every direction, 360 degrees around. Think of your hips as a lariat circling around your knees, which remain stationary.

These movements may feel awkward to you at first. Move past this feeling. The farther you can extend your pelvis in any given direction for each part of the circle, the better. The curve of your body can never be too deep or too round.

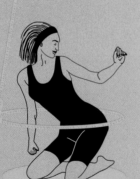

Circle ten times counterclockwise, then change direction for ten more circles.

TIME: 10 seconds per circle

body benefit:
Increasing mobility in the hip area is vital for maintaining locomotive abilities as we age. Movement of the pelvic girdle stimulates and massages the reproductive organs, keeping them healthy.

6 Tuck your butt and push your pelvis forward toward the wall in front of you. Allow your upper body to counter backward.

2 Begin making a wide, slow counterclockwise circle with your hips. Start by pushing your left hip out toward the left wall as far as you can.

3 Circle your hips to the rear as you inhale. Sweep your butt as far behind you as you can, arching your back and allowing your breasts to push forward to counter your hips.

4 Swing your hips slowly around to the right, pushing your right hip as far out to the right as you can.

5 Exhale as you circle your hips to the front.

TRANSITION Getting Up
Place your left foot on the floor in front of you. Pivot your body ninety degrees to the right as you place your left buttock down on your left heel. Raise your right knee and come into a crouch on both feet, then push your body up slowly—butt first—into a stand.

→

standing hip circles

These should be the biggest, roundest, most exaggerated circles your hips are capable of making. Do the opposite of everything women are usually taught: try to take up as much space as possible with your body, letting it reach ever farther past what you think its boundaries are.

TIME: 10–12 seconds per circle

body benefit:
The deeper you bend your knees, the wider the curve becomes and the harder your quads will work.

1 Stand with your feet a little more than hip-width apart. Bring your right hip toward the right wall.

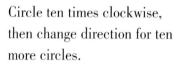

Circle ten times clockwise, then change direction for ten more circles.

5 Bring your hips back around to the right, pushing your right hip out toward the right as far as you can. Continue the circles. Don't lock your knees.

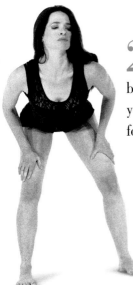

2 Begin making wide, slow, clockwise circles with your hips as you inhale. Stick your butt out as far behind you as you can, arching your back and allowing your breasts to come forward to counter your hips.

3 Swing your hips slowly around to the left, pushing your left hip as far out to the left as you can.

4 Exhale as you circle your hips to the front. Tuck your butt and push your pelvic bones out toward the wall in front of you. Allow your upper body to counter backward. Take as much time circling around front as you do around back.

Katherine's Hips

Katherine, thirty-five, grew up in an environment where women were frowned upon for wearing pants to church, to say nothing of letting their hips and butt stick out naturally. When she first came to my class, she had no idea what I meant when I told her to push her hip out as far as she could to the right—she simply had no concept of her body's true range of motion. At one point during her second class, I stood next to her, urging her to keep pushing her hip out farther and farther. Then, suddenly, her hip unlocked and she got it way out there. Her face lit up with a look of childlike wonder. From years of keeping her hips locked in a linear frame, the pathway of energy in her body had become blocked in the pelvic region like a kinked garden hose. She told me later that when she pushed her hip out and unkinked it, she felt a sudden rush. "It was like energy was flowing from the top of my head to the bottom of my feet for the first time in my life. And I felt like I was finally living in my entire body."

full body circles

In this move, your entire upper body moves like the arm of a windmill in a slow, huge circle perpendicular to the floor. Your head will counter the movement of your pelvis. Slow and deliberate movement is of utmost importance here to avoid getting dizzy.

TIME: 10–12 seconds per circle

sensual focus:
Focus on a single instrument in the music and allow your body to follow its path through the song.

1 Stand with your feet a little more than shoulder-width apart, with your knees slightly bent, your left hip pushed out to the left, and head dropped back.

Continue the circle five times, then reverse the direction and repeat.

6 Bring your torso upright as you inhale. Push your pelvis forward, and let your head fall back.

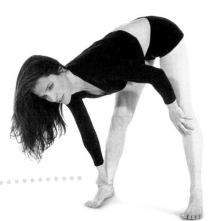

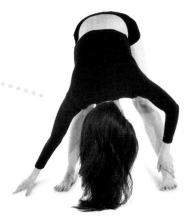

3 Exhale as you sweep your upper body down toward the floor, pushing your butt out to the back.

2 Begin making wide, slow circles with your upper body, counteracting its movement with your hips. Bring your upper body over to the right as your left hip pushes out to the left.

4 Sweep your upper body to the left as you bring your right hip out to the right.

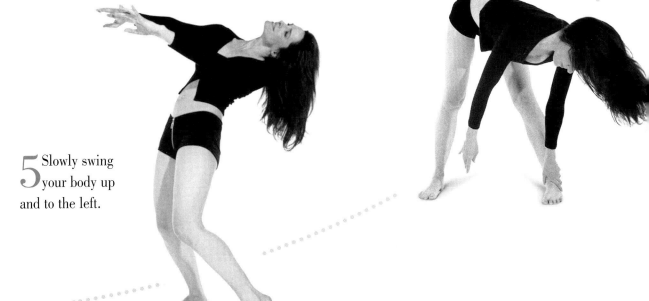

5 Slowly swing your body up and to the left.

butt circles

This move is a pure celebration of your best asset—in all its glory. Here, you focus the exaggerated movement in your butt. Butt circles give an amazing stretch to your lower back, and are a good exercise to come back to whenever you feel fatigue in your spine.

TIME: 5 seconds per circle

body/mind benefit:

Endorphins are naturally occurring neurotransmitters that resemble opiates—in fact, the word comes from the Greek, meaning "inner morphine." Times of high endorphin production include sex, exercise, and meditation. The S Factor combines all three of these. Studies have shown that increased endorphin production leads to greater heart health and lower stress levels, and may even prevent cancer. So the sense of well-being you feel during your workout does, in fact, correlate to real effects in your body.

1 Stand with your feet a little more than hip-width apart. Bend your torso slightly forward and place your hands on your knees. Arch your back.

RETURN TO STEP 2, with your butt back. Repeat clockwise nine times; then change directions for ten more circles.

5 Bring your butt around to the right.

2 Slowly begin making circles with your butt, resting your weight on your hands and keeping your upper body still. Inhale as you push your butt straight back as far as possible, keeping your back arched.

3 Move your butt around to the left.

4 Exhale as you tuck your butt forward and scoop your belly.

RIPPLE EFFECT

Hip work can be a profound experience for many women. My students are often surprised to find that they have a trove of sexual energy locked away in their hips and pelvis. Unlocking it can come as a revelation. The most common response in class is a giddy, irrepressible high. Students tell me stories about driving home from class in a blissful state. I have one student who was so ecstatic after her first class that she called every person in her Palm Pilot to tell them about this great new thing she'd discovered. One after another, they hung up on her. Her class had ended at eight. She's from England and it was three in the morning there. She didn't care and kept dialing away. Before you go to such lengths to tell the whole world about your new thing, try writing about it in your journal.

Occasionally, stronger emotions come up. Long-held memories, locked away in unused muscles in your hips and pelvic area, may surface and you may feel a tangible release of emotion—ranging from joy or surprise to sorrow or fear. I encourage you to laugh, cry, and work through your feelings in the movement and in your journal.

If you're feeling some apprehension, it may come from internalized judgments—a lifetime of inherited messages that the world you're entering is off-limits. You might have learned that "good girls" don't move this way and it may unnerve you to know that hidden within your good-girl façade or your mommy persona lurks a powerfully erotic person.

The Naked Truth

Look at the advertisements in any fashion magazine today and you'll see a gorgeous model standing, sitting, or lying in a sexually suggestive position with half of her clothes falling off. She looks ripe, inviting, devastating. Who wouldn't want to be her?

Now go to any strip club and you'll see a woman moving from one sexually suggestive pose to another, slowly peeling off layers of clothes. She looks ripe, inviting, and devastating, yet no one wants to be her.

What's the difference between these two women? Perception. Status. Money. The model has power and prestige, while the stripper has a bad reputation and maybe gets two hundred bucks—on a good night.

If you are experiencing feelings of shyness or discomfort about what you've been learning, take a moment to look around you. Almost every billboard, TV ad, and fashion magazine is filled with sexually suggestive images. These beautiful women are owning and exaggerating their sexuality. The prevalence of these images in the media says how acceptable, even desirable, society considers these sexy poses and dress.

Picture This

The following exercise should be done in a room without a mirror; it's designed to help you give yourself permission to be as overtly sensual as the glamorous models in magazines.

1. Pick up three or four fashion or entertainment magazines. Leaf through the pages and tear out pictures that strike you as sexy or erotic: half-clad women; women in provocative poses; women touching themselves sensually; women dressed, lit, or made up in ways that seem seductive to you.

2. Choose the three pictures you like best. Tape the photos up on the wall in front of you and study them carefully.

3. Spend ten minutes mirroring each picture—its overall theme, feeling, and attitude. As you turn and curve your body, let it morph from one picture into another. Repeat this morphing three times or until your body memory kicks in and you don't have to look at the pictures anymore. Remember to breathe into each pose.

In your journal, record your thoughts about the pictures and your feelings about doing the poses. Did it surprise you to discover just how prevalent these sexual images are?

Which of the images felt most "you" to you? Why?

Which felt least like you? Why?

Were you surprised at how easy or difficult it was to place your own body in similar poses?

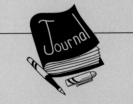

chapter three: coming out to

The S Factor movements are meant to mine something true and real within you—your organic, innate sexual nature. Will other people notice the change in you? Absolutely. Will you appear sexier to them? Perhaps. But sensuality—*real* sensuality—comes from the inside. It's not about acting sexy in some prescribed way. It's not about being Marilyn, Madonna, or Pamela.

play: stripper moves

It's about being yourself. Before you can show off the goods for someone else, you must become convinced that your goods are worth showing off. That's the goal of this chapter: to reveal to you the wonder and glory of your own beauty.

The following exercises are called Stripper Moves because they're the moves every stripper learns in the clubs. They are both seductive and provocative, but for now, think less about how they'll look to someone else and pay careful attention to your own sensual experience of each movement. Find enjoyment in the simplest gestures—your hand running over your belly, the arch of your back, the slow roll of your head. Think of each movement as a chance to lay claim to your body, to take pride in its curves and fullness and textures.

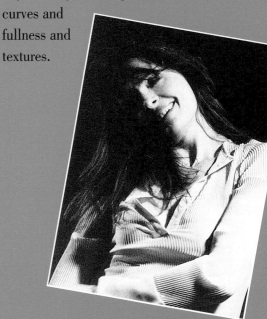

CATCH THE WAVE

The beat of a song relates to the rhythm and tempo as defined by the drum and bass; the wave is a slower, broader undercurrent that derives from the phrasing of the music. It's harder to catch at first, but with practice it becomes intuitive. The exercise below should help you to begin to identify the wave. In S Factor movement, you never want to move on the beat of the music (with a couple of exceptions, addressed later). Rather, you want to find that slower, subtler undercurrent and ride it like a wave.

Every song has a beat and a wave, but in most songs, one is more dominant than the other. Throbbing dance music and hard rock tend to have a more accessible beat, while slower, more melodic, less rhythm-driven songs have a more identifiable wave. The exercise below should help you to begin to identify the wave.

Put on Led Zeppelin's "D'yer Mak'er" or any hip-hop music and notice how the song is propelled by the powerful bass and drum. The wave trails underneath and behind the beat, but it's there.

Now put on Coldplay's "Clocks" and hear how the wave lives in the piano and the singer's voice. Close your eyes and you can almost see the wave of music coming at you.

To experience moving in this different way, put on something from the musical selections on the facing page and do some Inverted Spine Circles (page 8), following the beat of the music. Then slow your movement down. Slower, slower, as if you're stringing eight beats together in an arc. Close your eyes and imagine that your body is floating on the ocean, like a surfer waiting for a wave. When you feel the wave pick you up, go with it. Ride on top of it, let it curl under you and around you. If you feel yourself losing the wave, slow it down again, and wait patiently. You'll find it.

Living in the wave of the music instead of the beat gives *you* more power than the song.

"Music melts all the separate parts of our bodies together."

—Anaïs Nin

liquid cruise music

For the Stripper Moves section, I recommend wave-heavy music. Choose songs with melodies and words that speak to you on a personal level. Below are some of my own favorites:

Smashing Pumpkins, *Adore:* "To Sheila"

Smoke City, *Flying Away:* "Underwater Love"

This Mortal Coil, *It'll End in Tears:* "Song to the Siren," "Another Day"

Nick Cave and the Bad Seeds, *The Boatman's Call:* "Into My Arms"

Muddy Waters, *Folk Singer:* "My Captain," "My Home Is in the Delta," "Long Distance"

Miriam Makeba, *Mama Africa: The Very Best of Miriam Makeba* (Almost anything from this album)

Ryan Adams, *Gold:* "When the Stars Go Blue"

Indian sculpture of dancing woman, circa 10th–12th century A.D.

© NIMATALLAH / ART RESOURCE, NY

Origins of Erotic Dance

Though the exact date of origin of erotic dance is not known, it is well documented that rolling, undulating hip movements were not originally intended as titillation for men but rather as expressions of the female body's power to promote fertility in the land. In ancient matriarchal cultures, dance was performed by women and for women exclusively. Versions of the dance—in which the natural shape of a woman's body was reflected in movements that originated in the hips rather than the legs or feet— were practiced widely in nearly all ancient cultures, through the Middle East, Africa, India, and Asia. They were usually incorporated into rituals that united the religious with the sensual in fertility rites, wedding preparations, and birth rituals.

It was only later, beginning with the advent of the Judeo-Christian patriarchal culture about 2,000 years ago, that a rift between the spiritual and the sensual developed. Movements like belly dancing were labeled "erotic" and performed by women for men. This development turned what had once been a religious, celebratory female rite into a taboo practice that, in our culture, took the form of "stripping" with its "dirty" connotations.

peel up

This is the first step in the next several leg exercises. I use the word *peel* often in this book: it describes a type of movement that should remind you of a banana peel slowly coming away from the flesh of the fruit. Allow yourself to feel a slight resistance during this slow, deliberate movement.

TIME: 5 seconds

body benefit:
The Peel Up stretches the back of the legs (hamstrings) while increasing strength in the quadriceps, hips, and abdomen.

Note: *As you move through the leg work in the next few exercises, your legs may start to shake and feel weak. Persevere and the weakness will go away as you strengthen and stretch your body.*

1 Sit with your legs extended in front of you, knees slightly bent at different heights. Lengthen your feet.

4 Slowly straighten your legs, first the right, then the left, extending your toes toward the ceiling.

2 Rock back so that your weight rests on your left elbow. As you rock back, lift your right knee toward the ceiling, keeping your feet lengthened.

3 Rock onto your right elbow so that your weight rests on both elbows. As you do this, lift your left knee up, keeping your toes pointed.

Beginner Modification

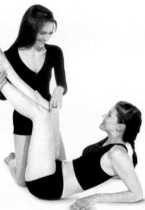

If this exercise is hard on your hamstrings, keep a slight bend in your knees and cross your ankles as you extend the legs upward.

fiddler

This movement reminds me of the way crickets rub their legs together to make music, or the way a violinist strokes her bow across the strings of her instrument. Keep these images in mind as the friction between your calves creates a resonance not unlike a strain of music.

TIME: 5 seconds for each foot

sensual focus:
As your ankle runs down your calf, focus on the smoothness of your skin.

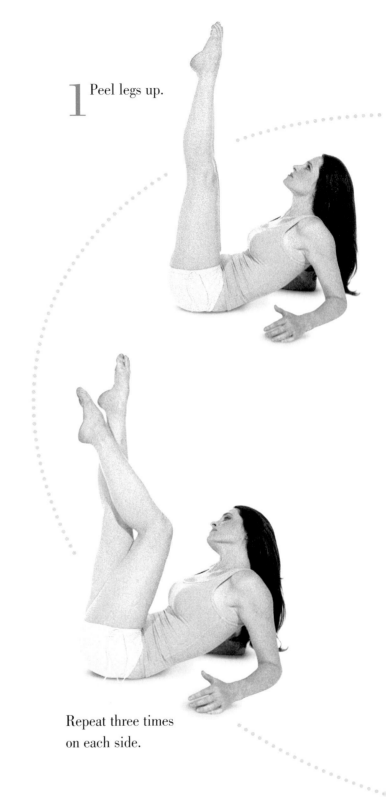

1 Peel legs up.

Repeat three times on each side.

2 Bending your left knee, slowly slide the inner edge of your left ankle down the inside of your right ankle and calf. Bring your left knee toward your right shoulder, keeping your feet lengthened. Slide your left foot back up your right calf and ankle.

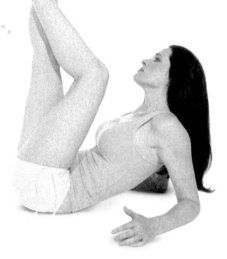

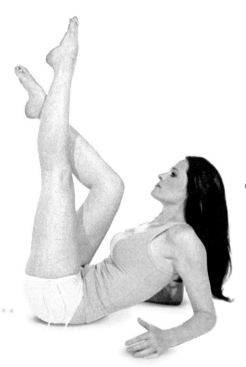

3 When your left leg has straightened up, slide your right ankle down the inside of your lower left leg, bringing the right knee in toward the left shoulder. Then slowly slide the right foot up again.

prance

The Prance shows off the beauty of your legs, the curve of the thighs and calves as they cut ever so slowly through the air. Focus on lengthening your legs all the way from the hip through the extended foot and pointed toe. Suddenly it will look as if you have those enviable "legs that go on forever." Remember to bring your knee in toward the *opposite shoulder* to get the most beautiful, curvaceous line of movement, as well as a more demanding workout on the abs.

TIME: 6 seconds per prance

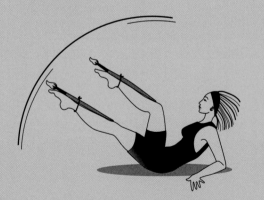

sensual focus: In the Prance, imagine that each foot is a paintbrush with which you are painting a huge, continuous arc across the ceiling, down the opposite wall, and across the floor.

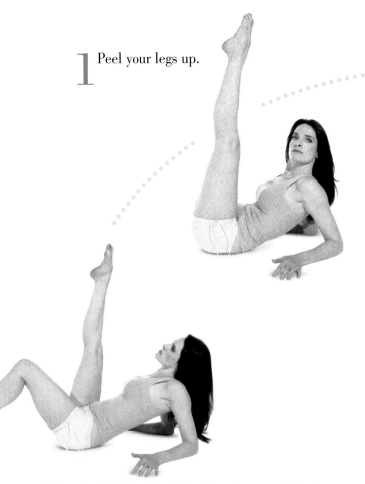

1 Peel your legs up.

7 When the left foot is within three inches of the floor, bend the left knee and bring it in toward your right shoulder. With an inhalation, begin to lower the right leg again. Continue for twenty strokes (if you can!).

6 As you exhale and lower the left leg toward the floor, begin to straighten the right leg up toward the ceiling.

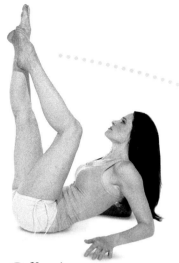

2 Keeping your right leg straight and foot lengthened, gently bend the left leg.

3 On an inhalation, slowly lower your straight right leg down toward the floor.

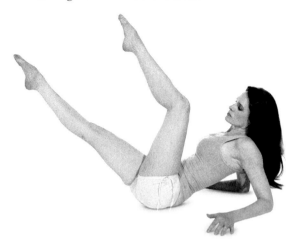

4 When your right foot is within three inches of the floor, straighten the left leg.

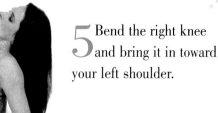

5 Bend the right knee and bring it in toward your left shoulder.

flirt

In the Flirt, you are drawing a semicircle in the air right down to your vulva, as though your pointed toes are gently guiding your awareness there. (Imagine that your lower right leg is the hand of a clock. Travel from 12, past 9, down to 6.)

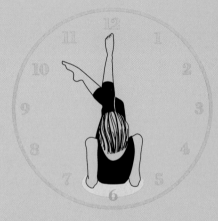

TIME: 5 seconds per flirt

sensual focus:
As you do this move, think of your lower leg as a warm knife cutting through a block of chocolate ice-cream cake, while keeping the movement slow and controlled.

1 Peel legs up. Cross your ankles so that your right leg is behind the left, keeping your legs straight and feet lengthened.

Repeat steps 2–6 three times. Then do four on the other side.

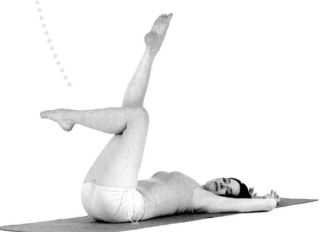

6 Do the same with your left leg. Allow it to pivot at the knee and make a semicircle to the right and down to the groin and back up.

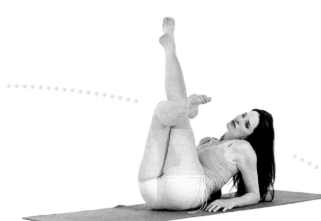

3 Continue the arc down to your groin (6 o'clock). Keep both feet lengthened.

2 Keeping your knees together, inhale as you bend your right knee, using your right foot to draw a counterclockwise semicircle to the left.

4 Exhale as you bring your right foot back up along the same route (from 6 to 9 to 12).

5 When your right foot reaches the top, cross it in front of your left, keeping your legs straight and feet lengthened.

leg splay

This move is all about being open. As you open yourself up completely, be aware that you are unabashedly celebrating the core of your femininity. If you're lying flat on your back, run your hands down the inside of your legs to your crotch. Take ownership of your body; you are staking your claim to what is rightly yours.

TIME: 15 seconds

sensual focus:

The key to this move is imagining resistance with each movement. When opening the legs, pretend that your ankles are encircled with a thick rubber band that you have to push against to pry your legs open. When closing your legs, imagine you have ten-pound weights hanging from each ankle.

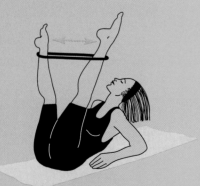

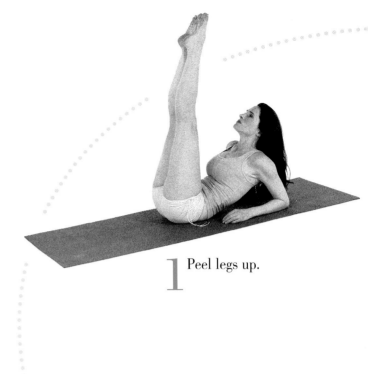

1 Peel legs up.

Repeat three times.
Remember to breathe.

5 Slowly pull your legs back up and together, keeping feet lengthened.

2 Inhale as you open your legs slowly, feet lengthened. Exhale.

Alternate Steps 2 and 4

We're all built differently, so don't worry if your legs don't open as far as you'd like. Lie with your back on the floor and peel legs open only as wide as you can. Breathe deeply into the stretch.

4 Exhale as you straighten your legs and lengthen your feet.

3 Inhale as you flex your feet and bend your knees (as in a plié).

bridge grind

This is a very sexy, slightly naughty variation of the Hip Circle. Remember to breathe through the movement.

As an alternative, try the Bridge Pump. Rather than make hip circles, pump your hips straight up and down, ten times. You can pump slowly for the best possible stretch and workout, or you can speed up for a raunchy effect during a routine.

TIME: 7 seconds per circle

sensual focus:
Imagine that you are lying inside a tube: the circles you make should take your pelvis around the inside surface of the tube.

1 Lie on your back with your knees bent, your feet flat on the floor slightly wider than hip-width apart and your arms resting at your sides along the floor.

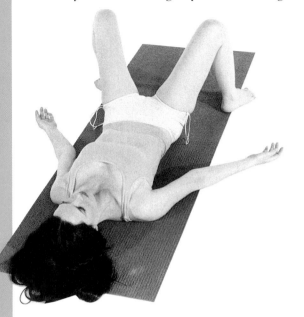

Repeat five times. Switch directions and do five more circles.

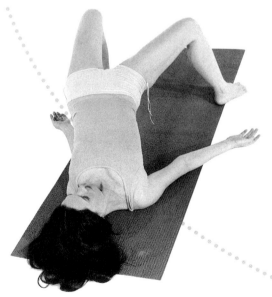

5 Continue the circle with your hips, to the left and back up toward the ceiling. As your hips come up, exhale.

2 Exhale as you slowly lift your hips off the ground and roll up your spine, vertebra by vertebra, until all of your body's weight is on your shoulder blades and feet. Push your hips up toward the ceiling.

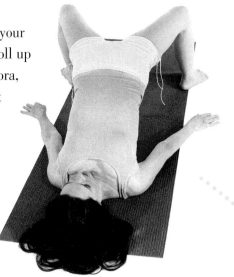

Counter-Stretch

After the fifth roll in the opposite direction, come back to the top and push your hips up as far toward the ceiling as you can, while tightening your butt. Inhale and hold for a couple of seconds. Exhale as you gently roll down your spine, vertebra by vertebra. Bring your knees up to your chest to stretch out the lower back for a couple of deep breaths.

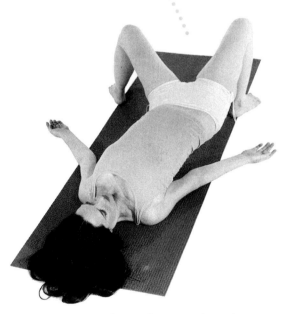

4 Inhale as your hips sweep down toward the floor, almost touching it.

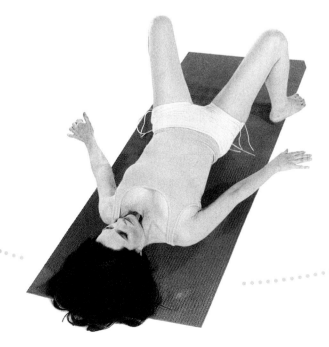

3 Begin to draw a large circle with your hips to the right and down.

crossover/ side goddess

Though technically a transition to side moves and Goddess poses, the Crossover is a useful move in its own right because it provides an important stretch to the abdominal and back muscles. Your body will thank you for it after the previous few exercises. The position you end up in is the Side Goddess.

Do the Crossover into a Side Goddess on each side to get an equal stretch. (That is, cross your left leg in front of your right, and twist over onto your right side.)

sensual focus:
The Crossover is a perfect opportunity to view your body at its best. The twist in your torso will exaggerate your curves. And even if you don't usually think of yourself as voluptuous, you will be in this pose.

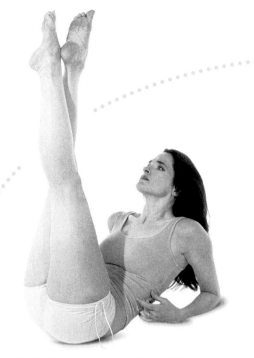

1 Lying on your back, peel legs up. Cross the right leg in front of the left, keeping both knees slightly bent and feet lengthened.

2 Imagine your right knee is being pulled over toward the left. The right leg will pull your whole body over to the left side.

3 Lower your legs slowly down to the floor on your left side, keeping both elbows on the floor as long as possible.

4 Let the twist in your torso pull your right shoulder off the floor and your upper body onto your left side. You may rest on your left elbow, with the right knee bent and crossed over the slightly-less-bent left leg. This position is called the Side Goddess.

side leg peel

It's more important with the Side Leg Peel to lift your knee as close to your shoulder as possible than to get your leg straight. This move reminds me of the unfurling of a flower petal in time-lapse nature photography, where each petal slowly extends itself outward as if taking a luxurious morning stretch.

TIME: 20 seconds per side

body benefit:
This movement works the superficial as well as the deep gluteus muscles. The stretch to the back of the legs (hamstrings) helps maintain pelvic alignment as well as blood flow to the legs. Opening the back side of the legs can also help alleviate tension on the sciatic nerve.

1 Lie on your left side in the Side Goddess position.

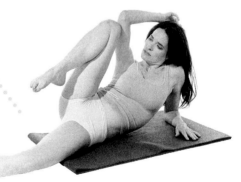

Lower the right knee to the floor as you **RETURN TO STEP 1.**
   Turn onto your right side and do steps 2–5 with the left leg.

6 Exhale as you bend your right knee and bring your pointed toe back down toward your left inner thigh.

2 Inhale as you lift your right knee as far as possible toward your right shoulder, keeping your toe pointed toward your left inner thigh.

3 With your hand on your calf or ankle, slowly extend the right leg toward your head. Go only as far as is comfortable.

4 Inhale and bring your straight leg down to the floor in front of your face. Keep your foot lengthened.

5 Bring your leg back up and exhale as you slowly trail your right hand down the inside of the right leg toward the crotch and back.

Beginner Modification

Lie flat on the floor and bend your knee as you draw your leg toward your head. The bent knee looks just as sexy.

TRANSITIONS

Transitional moves are as important as the individual moves because they bring the exercises together into one continuous, flowing routine.

Your goal should be to keep your movements fluid throughout the workout, never breaking the flow between exercises. Think of the routine as a long paragraph written in script with your hand never leaving the page.

Just as with the regular moves, the key to transitions is to do them *slowly*. Physically, imagine you are submerged in water—feel the simultaneous resistance of the water against your limbs and the weightlessness of the smallest movement. Or try to envision what you look like when you are just waking up—stretch into each movement with the same hazy feeling that you try to shake off with that morning cup of coffee. Ideally, a transition will be as deliberate, slow, and delectable as the movements it links together. To make a transition sensual, apply the same principles that you do in all S Factor movement (see page 12).

Ultimately, you will find that you can do anything sensually and deliberately. No movement will be extraneous or utilitarian; everything you do, even if you're walking across the floor or turning around, can and should be turned into a "stripper move" in its own right. It's all in the stretch and curve of your body. Like the swoop of a bird in flight or the graceful glide of a stingray, the transition should be indivisible from the movement.

In addition to the Belly Roll (facing page), below are some useful transitions to get from one S Factor move to another.

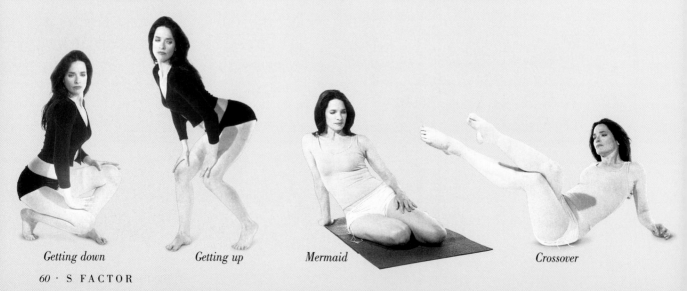

Getting down   *Getting up*   *Mermaid*   *Crossover*

belly roll

This is an essential transition between Side Leg Peels or from a Crossover into a Cat Pounce. Remember, though, that no matter how simple the move is, it should involve the greatest possible stretch, slowness, and sensuality you can bring to it.

1 Lie on your left side.

2 Slowly, on an exhalation, leading with your belly, roll onto the front of your body.

3 You may end the Belly Roll here, or go into a Cat Pounce (next exercise), or continue to roll up onto your right side.

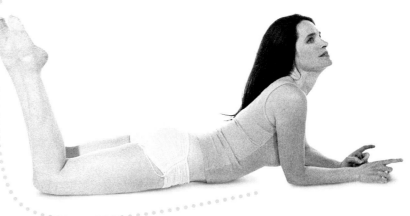

cat pounce

You often see a cat in this posture—somewhere between a stretch and a pull-back before pouncing on a toy or prey. The key to the Cat Pounce is to let your entire body be pulled up by your butt, as though you're being airlifted by a helicopter connected to a rope around your hips.

TIME: 8 seconds (minimum)

sensual focus:
As you do the Cat Pounce, pause for a few seconds with your chest resting on the mat and your butt high in the air. Notice how it feels to allow your butt to take up all that space: a powerful and defiant posture, like mooning the world. It goes against every puritanical, antisexual bone in your body. And that's why it rocks!

body benefit:
Like a garden hose, the spinal cord needs to be free of kinks. When there is an imbalance between the abdominal and back muscles, the vertebral column is pulled out of proper alignment. This stretch helps to realign it.

1 Lie flat on your belly with your legs about hip-width apart and your left cheek resting on the floor. Keep your elbows bent with your hands on the floor next to you and your feet lengthened.

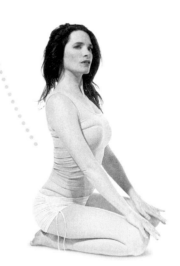

6 Keep the arch in your back throughout, butt pushed out behind you, and chest pushed forward as you rise.
Finish in a kneeling position.

2 Arch your back and inhale as you push your butt straight up toward the ceiling, using your abdominal muscles and arms to push yourself up. As your butt rises, slide your chest back toward your knees.

3 All of your weight should now be on your chest, face, and knees—not on your hands. You should be able to lift your arms off the floor and hold the position.

5 Push your body up onto your knees, allowing your chest and face to come up off the floor.

4 Lift your butt up and back. Keep your chest on the floor as long as possible.

picasso arch

This pose resembles a Picasso painting: a viewer will see only pieces of your body, arranged in a kind of cubist composition—a breast, part of a face, a hand, a belly, a butt. It's challenging to hold the pose, but if you can stay in it for about 30 seconds, you'll get the maximum benefit.

body benefit:

This move opens the thoracic cage (the chest), which may relieve asthma and other respiratory disorders and gently massages the front side of the heart. It makes the back and hips supple and opens the pelvic region. Allowing the head to fall back increases blood flow to the brain, which keeps those synapses firing. All in all, it's a kick-ass pose.

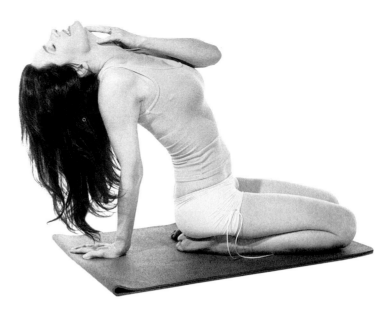

BEGINNER ARCH

Sit on your feet with your knees about hip-width apart. Place your right hand on the floor behind you, about a foot back from your feet. Keeping your butt on your feet, inhale and arch your back, pushing your breasts out in front of you while you support yourself on your right hand.

Touch Exercise

Let your head slowly roll back. With a full exhalation and inhalation, let your left hand travel down your body, starting at the top of your head and coming down to your crotch. Exhale as you slowly come back up to a sitting position.

INTERMEDIATE ARCH

Place your right elbow on the floor behind you, about a foot and a half behind your feet, with your palm on the floor. Supporting your weight on your elbow, exhale and arch your back up, allowing your head to fall back.

ADVANCED ARCH

Place your right hand behind you on the floor, about a foot behind your feet, with your fingers pointing toward the back wall. Inhale and arch your back while you support your weight on your right hand, lifting your butt off your feet and pushing your pelvis as far forward as you can.

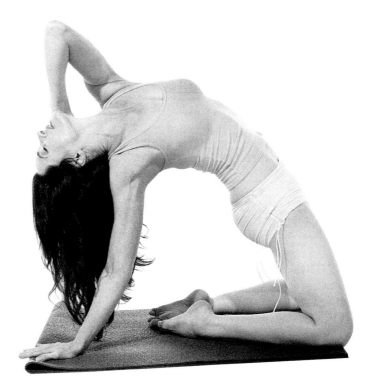

hump

This is a stylized simulation of riding a horse—an activity that, as we all know, is loaded with sexual connotations. It can be done quickly, with a lot of bounce, for an unsubtle effect, or slowed down to a more demure (and quad-torturing) speed, like the difference between a fast trot and a slow canter.

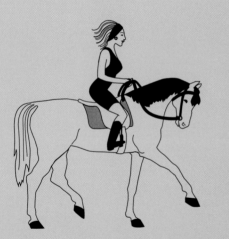

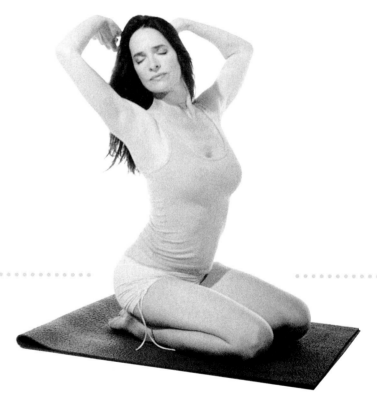

1 Sit on your feet, with your knees about hip-width apart.

Ride Your Emotions

Embrace and move through whatever emotion you bring with you to your workout. Once, a student arrived at class feeling awful. She had just come from a business meeting where she'd felt humiliated and disempowered. As she started working out, she filled her movements with the intense anger she was feeling and exorcised it through her body. It was spectacular to see. Her entire body morphed into an erotic warrior. Trust your body; it knows better than you do what it needs.

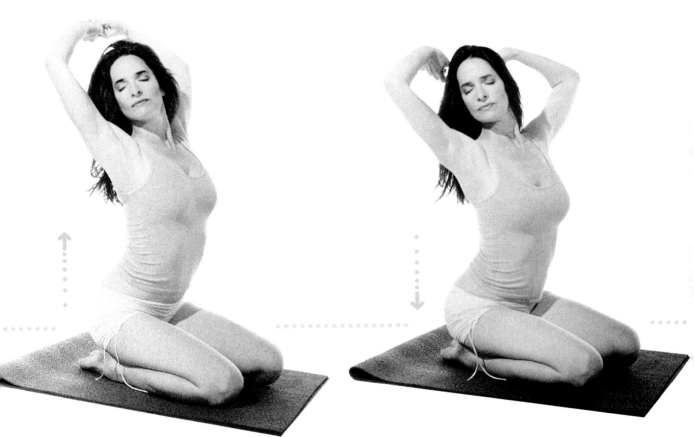

2 Arch your back, pushing your breasts out toward the wall in front of you, your butt toward the wall behind you. Rest your hands on your thighs, or hold them up above your head flirtatiously, with your elbows bent.

3 Bounce your upper body straight up and down rapidly, keeping your abs tight and the arch in your back pronounced, 10–15 times. Do not move your pelvis back and forth or hips from side to side; the only motion should be a straight up-and-down bounce of the torso.

pump

The most important thing to remember when doing the Pump is that your hips and pelvis don't move back and forth at all. Rather, your entire torso moves up and down on a 45-degree diagonal. It helps to keep your back arched and make sure your right hand is out to your side rather than behind you.

TIME: 3 seconds per Pump

visual focus:
Imagine that your entire torso is moving up and down on a skewer that's pointing at a 45-degree angle to the floor.

1 Sit on your feet, with knees together. Place your right hand on the floor, about a foot away from your right hip. Transfer your weight to your right hand.

Do five Pumps. Repeat on the other side.

4 When your left thigh is about parallel to the floor, exhale and lower your body back down to the floor.

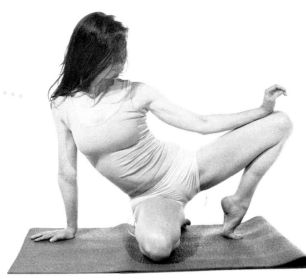

2 Lift your left knee off the floor and point it out to the left, coming up onto the ball of your left foot. (Your knees should be at a 90-degree angle to each other: the right knee pointed ahead, the left straight out to the left.) Arch your back and put your left hand on your left thigh.

45°

3 Arch your back, and with your left leg, push your torso up and to the right while supporting yourself with your right arm. Your hips should not move from side to side or front to back.

sitting body circles

A more advanced and challenging version of the Inverted Spine Circle (page 8), this movement requires more muscle control and balance. Let your head lead and your body will follow. It's an intimate move that brings your focus back to your center.

TIMING: 10 seconds per circle

sensual focus:
Relax your mouth and jaw as you focus on the tickle of your hair on your neck, shoulders, or across your face.

1 Sit on your feet with your knees together.

Do ten circles; then reverse direction and repeat.

6 Exhale as you scoop your belly and bring your head back around to the front.

5 Circle your head and upper torso to the left.

2 Exhale as you scoop your belly and curve your spine toward the wall behind you. Don't collapse over your lap; rather imagine you are cradling a basketball in your lap.

3 Circle your head and upper torso to the right.

Beginner Modification

When bringing your head around to the back in step 4, put your hands on the floor behind you.

4 Inhale as you sweep your head and shoulders around to the back, arching your back and pushing your chest out in front of you. For balance, extend your arms out in front.

pelvic grind

These are mini hip circles that you do while sitting on your feet. The only part of your body that you actually move is your pelvis, which will cause an undulation of the spine and head. Be aware of how your entire body is set in motion by even the smallest movement of the pelvis. Allow your spine and head to follow the flow of your pelvic circles.

TIME: 6–8 seconds per circle

sensual focus:
As your body moves, feel your chest and upper body pushing through thick air, as if it were stirring a vat of hot fudge.

1 Sit on your feet, with your knees about hip-width apart. Inhale as you push your butt out to the back, arching your back. Begin making clockwise circles with your pelvis, leaving your hands on your knees.

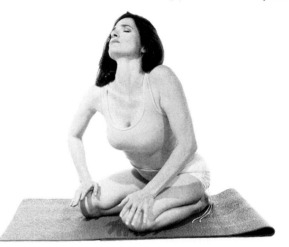

RETURN TO STEP 1.
Continue to circle, letting your spine, head, and neck be moved by your pelvic rotations. Do ten circles; then reverse direction and repeat for ten more.

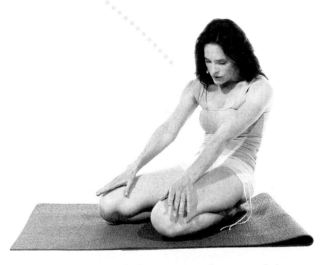

2 Circle your pelvis around to the left, letting your spine counteract the motion by pushing out to the right.

3 Exhale as you push your pelvis forward, allowing your spine to push out toward the back.

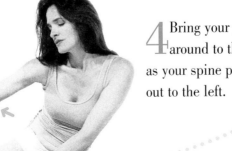

4 Bring your pelvis around to the right as your spine pushes out to the left.

mermaid

This transition gets you from a kneeling position to a seated one, or vice versa, with the greatest economy of movement.

1 Kneel with your knees about hip-width apart.

2 Keeping the arch in your lower back, bring your upper torso slowly forward as you lower your right buttock down to the floor to the right of your feet.

3 From here, you may roll back onto your elbows for a Peel Up or come down on your right side into a Side Goddess (page 56).

RIPPLE EFFECT

Feeling like a stripper yet? Maybe not quite, but that inner sensual core is heating up. Once you've practiced these moves, you may find yourself gazing appreciatively at the curve of your ankle as you sit on the bus. Or you'll catch yourself admiring your collarbones and shoulders the next time you dry off after a shower. Your awareness of your body's beauty is heightened by each of the exercises in this chapter, and the effects will follow you out into the world.

It's a great feeling to bring into the boardroom the next time you have an important meeting. Knowing your own erotic beauty turns you into your own most powerful ally. You may find that you worry less about what people think. You will be less apt to dwell on your body's shortcomings. Confidence will be easier to find and harder to lose. Already you will feel changes in your body as you start to use muscles you may never have used before. And you will definitely be sore. Very sore.

S Factor Meditation

Before moving on, it's important to integrate your emotional and physical selves. The point of this meditation is to release the tension in your body and to bring your conscious mind and your sexual self together using the healing power of your hands. The meditation should feel both relaxing and energizing. It's something you can do anytime you need to, even when you're not doing a workout.

To make the meditation more relaxing, I recommend that you read these instructions into a tape recorder and then play them back as you do the meditation. (You'll want to fill in instructions for the opposite body part.)

1 Put on some slow, mellow music. Make sure you have enough to last 30 minutes or put your CD player on repeat.

2 Lie down on your mat. Take a deep, slow breath. Then exhale and release all your tension. Inhale and lift your left leg three inches off the ground and point it hard, tensing all the muscles in the leg. Hold it, tightening for five seconds. Then exhale, release your leg, and place it on the floor. Do the same with your right leg.

3 Inhale and tense your butt. Squeeze it as hard as you can, tensing every muscle, tight, tight, tight. Then exhale and release.

4 Inhale and tense your pelvic and vaginal muscles (the same muscles you use to stop urinating). Squeeze them for five seconds, then exhale and release.

5 Inhale and tense your abdominal muscles. Squeeze them, pushing your belly down into the mat as hard as you can for five seconds. Then release.

6 Push your chest and breasts up toward the ceiling, filling your lungs with air and expanding the rib cage. Hold your breath for a beat, then exhale loudly, letting your chest drop and your muscles relax. Raise and tense your shoulders, lifting them up to your ears, then let them drop on a release of breath.

7 Inhale and tighten your left hand into a fist, lifting your left arm off the mat a few inches while tensing every muscle in it. Hold for five seconds, then exhale and let it drop. Repeat with the right hand and arm.

8 Inhale and lift your head half an inch off the mat. Tense the muscles in your neck and head, then exhale and gently lower your head back down.

9 Squish your face up like a fist, tightening around your eyes, nose, mouth, and forehead. Make a prune face. Exhale and let it relax.

10 Inhale and tense your whole body, almost lifting yourself off the mat. Hold for five seconds, then exhale and release everything.

11 Take a deep, slow breath all the way down into your feet. Imagine you are filling your body with vibrating yellow light from the sun or the moon. Exhale all the stress of the day—the traffic, the kids, school, work, men. Keep taking these deep and cleansing breaths, filling your body with light as you inhale. Exhale your breath from any place that you are still holding tension.

12 Start to move your left hand over your body. Turn your brain off and allow your hand to roam until it finds the place where you feel your sexuality resides. When your hand finds that spot, let it lie there and breathe into it, filling that area with a ball of warm, vibrating yellow light.

13 Now bring your right hand onto your body. Let it roam until it finds the place in your body where your consciousness resides—it could be anywhere—your head, your heart, your back, your neck. When you find that spot, let your hand rest there. Inhale, filling the area with warm yellow light.

14 You now have one hand on the center of your sexual power and one hand on your consciousness. Then, like a child finger-painting, use your two hands to smear the yellow light between the two spots. Move your hands back and forth on your body so that the two spots become one spot of vibrating, colorful sexual consciousness. Paint the light over your entire body.

15 Lie still for as long as you need to, luxuriating in this radiance. When you're done, take your time, wiggling your toes and opening your eyes, and let yourself come back slowly to the present.

chapter four: the goddess

O kay. Let's face it. There's a touch of wickedness to what I'm teaching you. In addition to being a great workout, the S Factor offers some of the most alluring movements known to humankind. And yes, if it's done for a man, it will drive him insane with desire. Go figure.

rising

In all likelihood, you're still at the point where you're practicing these movements alone, for yourself. There's nothing wrong with that. I recommend that my students wait until they're confident doing the exercises in this book before dancing for their lover.

You may decide, like many of the women in my classes, that the S Factor is something personal and private that you will never share with anyone. Or you may at some point want to dance for your husband or boyfriend, or even a girlfriend, to share your new discovery.

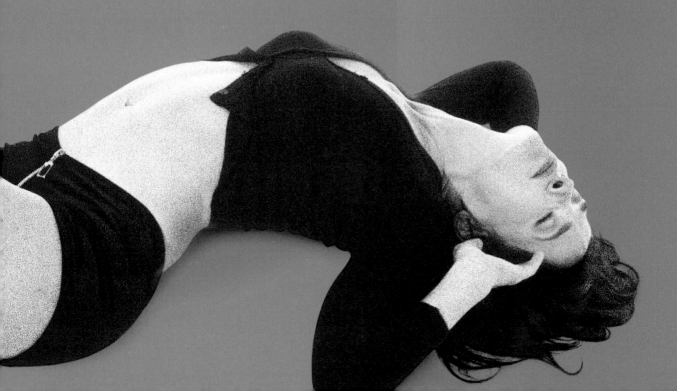

Either way, let's begin focusing some of your awareness outward. You will learn what moves arouse a man*, and you will develop confidence that your body has the power to rivet his attention. It's a mentality I often compare to that of a hunter, who must master the psychology and desires of her prey. The same applies to you in your stripper mode. Knowing how to command the gaze of your viewer will make your movement and striptease much more powerful.

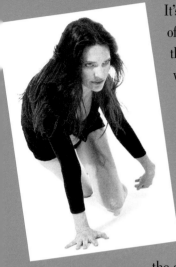

In the hunter's case, perfecting her art means using visual and other sensory lures to draw in her prey. In your case, it means knowing the sensory cues that arouse a man's interest and desire: beginning, of course, with the female form in all its glory—moving into, out of,

and around the beautiful Goddess poses. The positions and movements in this chapter are designed to exaggerate and show off the curves of your body. As you practice them, begin to tune your awareness to the shape your body creates, and the provocative effects of pushing your curves outward: curve turning into curve after curve.

bone pulse music

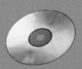 For the walk and crawl, try using more beat-heavy music, but remember to slip underneath the beat and ride the wave.

* **Lauryn Hill,** *The Miseducation of Lauryn Hill:* "Lost Ones"
* **Mary J. Blige,** *No More Drama:* "Family Affair"
* **White Stripes,** *Elephant:* "The Hardest Button," "Seven Nation Army"
* **R. L. Burnside,** *Come On In:* "It's Bad You Know," "Come On In" (parts 2 and 3)
* **Eminem,** *8 Mile* soundtrack: "Lose Yourself"

---

* *Although throughout this book I use the male pronoun when referring to the viewer, the S Factor is meant for anyone and everyone who wants to dance for a lover. Gay or straight, male or female, we can all stand to strip away inhibitions, to revel in our bodies, and to strut our stuff for our partners.*

goddess

The Goddess is a central pose in any S Factor routine—you can go into it during any point in your floor work and count on looking devastating.

1 Lie on your back with your feet lengthened and your arms slightly bent and out to the side.

2 Arch your back and push your chest up toward the ceiling, coming up onto the top of your head. As you do this, bend both knees at slightly different angles, keeping your feet lengthened. Breathe into this pose, keeping your abdominal muscles engaged to protect your lower back.

Beginner Modification

Rather than coming up onto your head, come up onto your shoulders with your back arched and your head flat on the floor.

writing goddess

This move takes the Goddess a step further, both physically and sensually. To get the fullest stretch and the most beauty out of this one, imagine you've got a big pillow under your shoulder blades.

sensual focus: Pay attention to every hill and valley on your body as you move your hands over your torso— your breasts, your stomach, your neck, your hips.

1 Lie on your back with your feet lengthened and your arms bent up and out to the side.

5 Continue to move your feet back and forth. Run your hands slowly and deliberately up and down your torso as you writhe. Remember to breathe and keep your abdominal muscles engaged.

2 Arch your back and push your chest up toward the ceiling, coming up onto the top of your head. Bend both knees at slightly different angles so that your right knee is a bit higher than the left.

3 Keeping your feet lengthened, slowly switch positions of your feet so that your left knee is higher than the right.

4 Keeping your motion continuous, switch your feet again as you bring your hands up onto your torso.

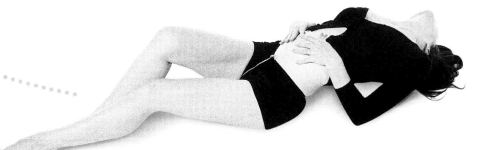

prancing
goddess

This is a more strenuous version of the Prance (see page 48), done in the Goddess pose. It's an advanced move, so work up to it by practicing the regular Prance and the Goddess. If you can master this move, you'll look incredible. Be aware that pivoting your hips ripples your body into a series of provocative positions, creating an undulation from your feet to the top of your head.

1 Start with the Writhing Goddess. The next time you bring your right knee up, lift your entire leg up until your right thigh is perpendicular to the floor.

5 Continue to pedal feet out and down, bringing each knee in toward the opposite shoulder, prancing your legs like a horse in slow motion. Breathe. Continue to prance, keeping back arched, for as long as desired.

2 Inhale and straighten (or nearly straighten) your right leg and lower it slowly down toward the floor. As you do this, bend your left knee and bring it up and in toward your right shoulder.

3 As your right leg approaches the floor, straighten (or nearly straighten) your left leg.

4 Lower your left leg down toward the floor and exhale. As you do this, bend your right knee and bring it up and in toward your left shoulder.

goddess rising

This transitional move coming out of or going into floor work builds extraordinary back and abdominal strength and looks devastatingly gorgeous.

TIME: 10 seconds

sensual focus:
Imagine there's a string attached to your breastbone and you're being pulled up by it.

1 Begin in the Goddess pose (see page 81).

4 Come up to a seated position. *Don't* curl or muscle your shoulders forward or pull your head up to rise. Your head should be the last part of your body to come up.

2 Using your arms and your abdominal and back muscles, push your chest farther up toward the ceiling.

3 Continue rising, chest-first, with your head following.

the s walk

The S Walk cannot be underestimated. It's one of the most important moves, the base around which you add all the subtle (or not-so-subtle) actions to your routine. It's how you express your power, your eroticism, your sensual self. It's also a lot of fun. Your S Walk transports you from the world of the ordinary into the realm of a sensual goddess.

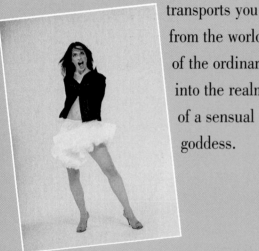

visual focus: A lioness stalking her prey steps stealthily, deliberately, with perfect control and economy of movement. She drags one paw in front of the other before placing it down. Her back undulates. Her long, cool gaze locks onto her prey. As you learn the Walk, keep this sublimely feline image in your mind's eye. Let the lioness enter your body through the music, through your senses. Imagine your body as something wild, yet perfectly controlled and lethal.

1 **Slow it down.** Walk in your normal, everyday walk a couple of times around the room. Then slow it *way* down so that you are walking at a quarter of your normal speed, inhaling on one stride, exhaling on the next.

2 **Cross over.** As you step, cross one foot over the other, (your left foot falling to the right of an imaginary center line, your right foot falling just to the left of it). This may feel awkward at first—that's okay. In time, the S Walk will feel natural, familiar, and delicious.

3 **Drag.** Become aware of your back foot. As you bring it forward, softly brush the floor with the top of your foot. Imagine you are walking on a beach and drawing a line in the sand with your toes.

4 **Fall into the hip.** Now as you step forward, *fall into your hip*. As your left foot becomes firmly planted on the floor, push your left hip out. Overstate the movement, allowing your body to fall even farther into your hips on each stride. Remember, it's a role you're playing, so have fun with it.

5 **Strut your stuff.** Arch your back. Open up your chest as you push your breasts up and out and your butt back and out, exaggerating your curves.

getting down

This is another essential transition step. In the Getting Down and Getting Up exercises, there is no such thing as too slow. That's why it's known as quad torture.

Practice, practice, practice will build up your quad muscles to make this move easier and more fluid.

sensual focus:
To keep it slow, imagine you are moving underwater and that you have to push your hips and butt out against the resistance the water creates.

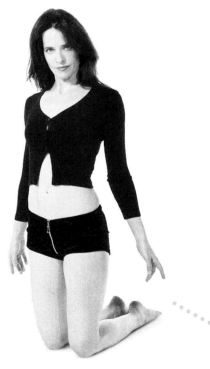

1 Stand with your feet slightly more than hip-distance apart. Circle your hips to the right.

5 Lower the left knee to the floor, then the right knee, so that you end in a kneeling position.

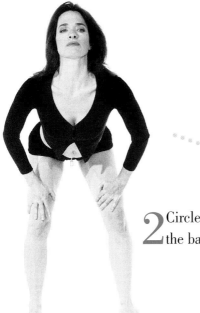

2 Circle your hips to the back.

3 As your hips come around to the left, bend both knees and begin to lower your butt.

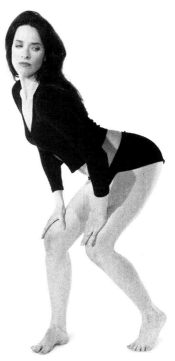

4 Come down to a half-squat with your right knee in the air and your left buttock resting on your left heel (your left foot should be in demipointe).

cat crawl

Watch a house cat move. It's provocative, but also a bit reserved and prim. That's the basic attitude for this first crawl. Cats don't use excess movement. They move only what is necessary to get where they're going in the most relaxed way possible. And sometimes they move just to feel themselves moving.

TIME: 2 seconds per stride

sensual focus:
Allow your back to undulate as you crawl. Relax your back muscles and drop your head, letting your shoulder blades rise and fall to their maximum height and depth. Exaggerate it.

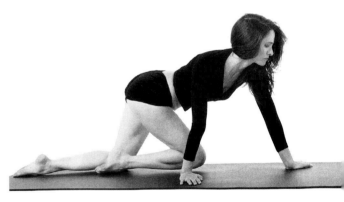

2 Slowly begin crawling, bringing your left hand and your right knee forward. Cross the right knee slightly over the left.

1 Get on your hands and knees, with your hands turned slightly out (right fingers pointing to the right, left fingers to the left).

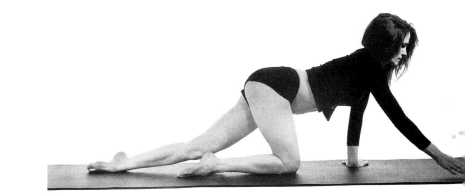

4 As you come onto each hand, fall into your shoulder, allowing the corresponding shoulder blade to rise up. As your weight comes down onto each knee, let your body weight relax into your hip.

3 Plant your left hand and right knee on the floor and bring the right hand and left knee forward.

wild cat crawl

When a lioness hunts, she first creeps silently toward her prey, staying hidden in the grass for as long as she can. Then, when she's advanced far enough, she lunges at the poor, unsuspecting creature in question. The Wild Cat Crawl mirrors this second phase—it's more overtly predatory and aggressive, coming in for the thrill.

sensual focus: Be aware of how this movement makes you feel more sexually aggressive. As you lock your gaze on "him" (even if it's just an empty chair or a mirror), notice how predatory you feel.

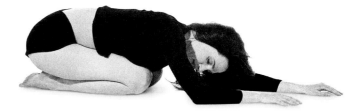

1 Crouch on the floor, sitting on your haunches, with your hands on the floor in front of you.

3 Reach your right hand and right knee as far forward as you can while keeping your left hand and knee stationary.

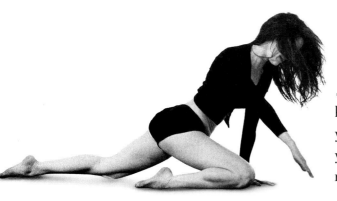

2 Raise your body up onto your hands and knees as you begin to bring your right knee and right hand forward.

5 Simultaneously bring the left knee and hand as far forward as you can, keeping your right hand and knee stationary.

4 When doing the Wild Cat Crawl in a strip routine, bend your head down to show off your rippling back.

getting up

In this transition, you may position yourself with your butt, your front, or your side to your viewer; any way gives a great show, especially when done oh-so-slowly. If you are feeling wobbly at any point, steady yourself by putting the tips of your fingers on the floor.

Both the Getting Up and Getting Down moves are easier if you're wearing 6-inch platforms.

sensual focus:
When my students do this movement, I sometimes suggest they do it as though they're thinking, "Oh, it's *soooo hard* getting up!" This slows down the transition and adds a little edge of petulance that's undeniably sexy.

1 Kneel on your mat. Bring your left knee up and forward and raise your foot into a demipointe (like you're proposing).

Repeat on the other side.

7 When your legs are nearly straight, bring your torso upright, keeping your back arched. You can swing your hips around into a standing Hip Circle.

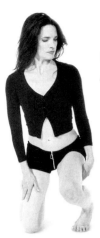

2 Pivot 90 degrees to the right with your right knee.

3 Sit your left buttock down on the heel of your left foot (still in demipointe).

4 Now bring your right knee up so you are in a full squat up on the balls of your feet, knees about shoulder-width apart. Put your hands on your knees.

5 Keeping your chest out, push against your knees to bring yourself to a standing position.

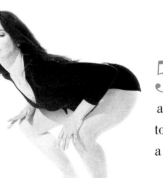

6 As you straighten your legs, push your butt out and back. Arch your back, and push your chest out and up.

TRANSITION **Wall Work**
As the name suggests, the next portion of the workout is devoted to elements that are done against a wall. The wall, like the pole later on, is an anchor whose support allows you to increase your stretches even farther. *97*

frisk

Think, "Ma'am, put your hands on the car." The inspiration for the name of this movement is the stance of being searched by a police officer. It's a hot image, endlessly played out in sexual fantasies the world over. But this is hardly a submissive movement—as you'll surely see when you give it a try.

TIME: 4 seconds

body benefit:
This is a killer hamstring stretch that makes your legs look luxuriously long and strong. In addition, stretching the chest in this way engages the muscles that support the vertebral column— excellent for your posture.

1 Stand about 2½ feet away from the wall, with your feet a little more than hip-distance apart. Place both hands on the wall in front of you and go up on your tiptoes.

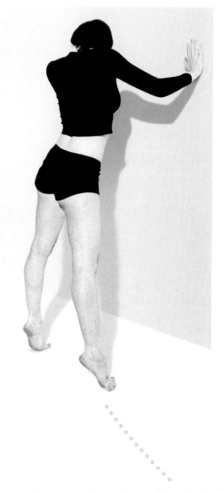

Reverse direction and circle back around to the right. Repeat five times.

2 Slowly circle your hips to the right, keeping your hands against the wall and your back arched.

4 Circle your hips around to the left (your torso will rise a bit here). Maintain the arch in your back and keep your butt pushed out.

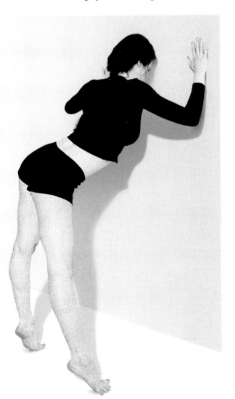

3 Circle your hips to the back, allowing your torso to push down toward the floor. Let your head drop down, relaxing your neck. Imagine that your back is a tabletop; try to keep it flat and parallel to the floor.

brain
massage
turn

A variation on the Brain Massage (see page 22), this is a beautiful transition that stimulates the follicles in the scalp, including the ones at the back of your head that you couldn't reach in the floor Brain Massage. Keep your breath flowing throughout the turn. If you find this exercise difficult, you may lean on your shoulder, or on your shoulder and head, as you pivot your body.

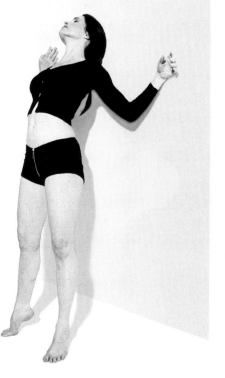

1 Begin in the same position as the Frisk (see page 98), about 2½ feet from the wall, up on your tiptoes. Place both hands on the wall in front of you.

Repeat, pivoting to the other side.

2 Lean your forehead against the wall.

3 Without letting your head lose contact with the wall, begin to pivot your body, using your hands against the wall for support.

4 Continue massaging your scalp, pivoting until your back is to the wall.

wall hip circles

This is a version of the Standing Hip Circles (see page 32) in which you can get an even greater range of motion by using the wall as support. It's a confident, "I know my worth" kind of move.

sensual focus:
As you circle your hips, allow your hands to wander teasingly up and down your torso. When your hips are pushed all the way forward, it's a great opportunity to play with the top of your pants or skirt. Pull and tug as if you're just aching to get out of them.

1 Stand with your back to the wall with your legs about 2 feet from it. Lean your back, shoulders, and head against the wall. Exhale and push your pelvis forward as far as you can.

Tucking your butt, circle the hips around to the front as you **RETURN TO STEP 1.** Continue the circles in one direction for five rounds and then repeat in the opposite direction.

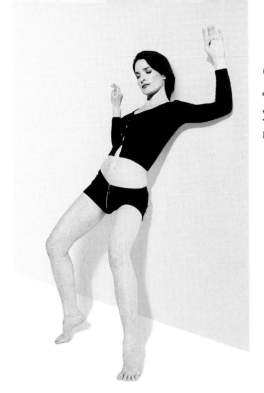

2 Start to circle your hips in a clockwise direction, keeping your knees bent and pushing your right hip as far to the right as you can.

3 Inhale and circle your hips and butt around to the back so they sweep against the wall you're leaning on. Keep your back arched.

4 Bring your hips around to the left, keeping your knees bent and pushing your left hip as far out to the left as you can.

wall slide

This move is a useful transition from the wall down to the floor. The effect should be that of your body slowly dripping down toward the floor like honey. So make the Wall Slide slow and smooth.

body benefit:
The Wall Slide is a serious workout for the quads, particularly when done with the advanced modification (right).

sensual focus:
This is a great moment in your routine to confront your viewer. Meet his gaze and nail him with your eyes as you slide down the wall.

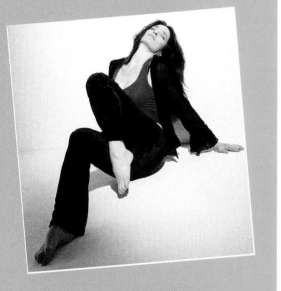

1 Stand with your back against the wall, with your feet shoulder-width apart and about a foot and a half from the wall, in demipointe.

2 Arch your back so that the only parts of your body resting on the wall are your head, butt, and shoulder blades. Use your abs to support your back and breathe into the abdominal stretch.

Advanced Modification: Wall Pump

In step 3, as you slide down, stop at the point where your quads are parallel to the floor and then push yourself back up almost to the top. Then lower again to the "sitting" position, then up again. Repeat as many times as you can.

5 End in a crouching position with knees bent at slightly different angles.

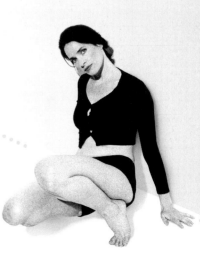

3 Slowly and smoothly, bend your knees and slide down the wall, keeping your shoulders and butt in constant contact with the wall.

4 As you approach a full crouch, you may put your hands on your knees for support. Remember to keep your back arched, abs tight.

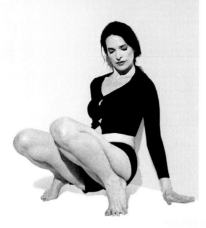

1 Do a Wall Slide down to a crouch on the floor.

A continuation of the Wall Slide, this is a modification of the Peel Up done when going from the wall to the floor. It can also be done against a pole. Take your time. Keep your movement slow and deliberate.

2 Place your hands on the floor next to your hips. Extend your right leg along the floor as you scoot your butt about a foot forward from the wall.

3 Lower your back to the floor, propping your head against the wall (as if it's a headboard). Begin to peel your legs up one at a time.

4 End with your arms outstretched to either side, your head against the wall and your legs peeled up and bent at slightly different angles.

RIPPLE EFFECT

Look in the mirror. Do you see a light behind your eyes? Do you have a mischievous feeling, like someone who has a secret? You do have a secret—you're feeling your own power. It's a power that will change the way you walk, the way you talk to others, the way you carry your body through life. I've seen it happen with my students. Within a couple of weeks, quiet, shy women who made every effort to take up as little space as possible were coming to class with a sparkle in their eyes, greater creativity in their work, renewed energy, more youthful demeanors, and a cocky attitude about their bodies. You, too, may find that you feel stronger, leaner, and more energetic. Your clothes fit more loosely and you spring out of bed in the morning after hitting the snooze button only once instead of your usual eight times.

One of my students, a 38-year-old mother of four, held her body curved in on itself like the letter C: weighted down at the shoulders, concave at the belly. After practicing the movements and her S Walk, pushing her butt and breasts out, opening her chest and heart, her energy has changed: she glows, exudes joy, and walks around in—I kid you not—what looks like the body of an 18-year-old.

Another change that began to occur among my students—perhaps you've noticed it, too—is that they find they're less apt to judge other women. Rather than feeling jealous or competitive, they appreciate and celebrate the beauty and sensual power they see in others. There's a reason for that: when you feel your own power, you don't have to be jealous of others. When you own and love and understand your body, you don't wish it looked like someone else's. When you realize just how strong women are, you can't help but give them props for it.

While practicing the moves in this chapter, you may have started to feel a bit like a goddess yourself. All of which begs the question, what kind of goddess are you? Take the fun "Goddess Quiz: What's Your Erotic Personality?" on the following page and see if you're a sultry, underworld creature or a blithe spirit of the Spring.

What's Your Erotic Personality?

To enhance your S Factor experience and bring your erotic creature further out of hiding, you need to continue exploring. What does she like to do? What kind of man is she drawn to? Who is she? Take this quiz, tally up your answers, and find out more about her.

1. It's Sunday and the whole afternoon stretches before you. What do you do?

a. Practice my kickboxing
b. Watch *To Kill A Mockingbird* again
c. Go for a swim in the lake
d. Go for a hike
e. Do the wild thing all day long— who needs hobbies?
f. Hang out with the kids and veg

2. What do you look for most in a man?

a. Someone with whom I can have a good knock-down, drag-out brawl
b. Someone who understands my moods
c. Someone I can take dancing
d. Someone who takes care of all the stuff, like bills and travel arrangements
e. A sexual stallion
f. A man who loves to work with his hands

3. Which book title most accurately represents your personality?

a. *The Woman Warrior*
b. *Notes from the Underground*
c. *A River Runs Through It*
d. *Lolita*
e. *The Joy of Sex*
f. *The Good Earth*

4. If your house was on fire, what would you save (after family and pets)?

a. My favorite combat boots
b. My diary/journal
c. Oh, come on—the house isn't going to burn down!
d. My childhood teddy bear

e. My vibrator
f. My family photo albums

5. If you were a cat, what kind would you be?

a. Alley cat
b. Black panther
c. Cheetah
d. Kitten
e. Cat on a Hot Tin Roof
f. Lioness

6. What's your dream vacation?

a. An African safari
b. Camping in Death Valley
c. Hawaiian rain forest
d. Disneyland at midnight
e. Paris
f. A dude ranch

7. Your dream vehicle would be:

a. A vintage Harley
b. The Batmobile
c. A yacht
d. A Jeep
e. A Lamborghini
f. An SUV

8. Your favorite color is:

a. Purple
b. Black or gray
c. Blue
d. Pink
e. Red
f. Green

Answers

*Add up your answers, and find which letter (**a–f**) shows up most often. If you have an even split—say, four **a**'s and four **d**'s—you might be a wonderful hybrid of two goddess types.*

a *answers*

THE HUNTRESS/WARRIOR

You're a fierce, assertive woman who doesn't back down from a challenge and usually gets what she wants.

Possible goddesses:

ARTEMIS/DIANA *(Greek/Roman):*
  Goddess of the Hunt
PINGA *(Native American): Huntress*
BADB *(Celtic): Goddess of War*

b *answers*

THE DARK SOUL

You're deep, moody, complex, intelligent, and powerful. Sure, you can be a handful. But what a handful! And talk about sexy.

Possible goddesses:

PERSEPHONE *(Greek): Goddess of the Underworld*
ERESHKIGAL *(Mesopotamian):*
  Goddess of the Underworld
HOLDA *(Norse): Goddess of Winter*
DURGA *(Hindu): Lady of Destruction*

c *answers*

THE WATER SPRITE/DANCER

You're generally lighthearted, but your waters run deep. You love to swim and dance—you're always the first one in the pool or to swivel your hips when the music starts.

Possible goddesses:

GANGA *(Hindu): Cleansing Stream*
OYA *(African): Lady of the River*
AMENOUDUME *(Japanese): Goddess of Dance*
YEMANJA *(South American): Mistress of the Sea*

d *answers*

THE NATURE CHILD

Eternally young at heart, you delight in play and pleasure. You love nature, dawn, and springtime; you are the light of your loved ones' lives, and you know it.

Possible goddesses:

OSTARA *(Norse): Goddess of the Springtime Festival*
LALITA *(Hindu): Playful Child*
CHASCA *(South American): Lady of the Dawn*
CERRYDWEN *(Celtic): Goddess of Nature*

e *answers*

THE SEXPOT

You're a hot one. You smolder, sizzle, seduce. You love being romanced and you expect to be well taken care of—in bed and out.

Possible goddesses:

APHRODITE/VENUS *(Greek/Roman):*
  Goddess of Love
FREYJA *(Norse): Seductive Sex Goddess*
HINE MOA *(Oceanic): Passionate Princess*
LILITH *(Mesopotamian): First Wife and equal of*
  Adam/Seductress

f *answers*

THE EARTH MOTHER

A nurturer and a homemaker, you're more than just a soccer mom; you're a queen among goddesses, the highest in the pantheon. Your strength is the deepest kind, drawn from the earth itself.

Possible goddesses:

GAIA *(Greek): Earth Mother*
HSIWANG MU *(Chinese): Queen Mother*
ISIS *(Egyptian): Mother Goddess*
MAKA *(Native American): Mother Earth*

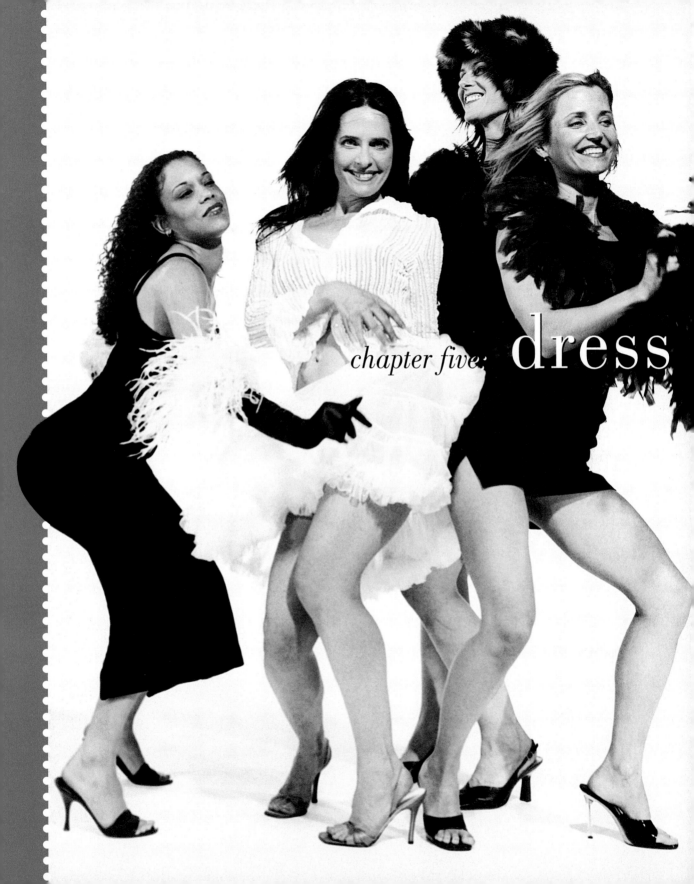

chapter five: dress

You can do a delectable strip out of absolutely any type of clothing. I have one student who wears nothing but a black evening gown and a strand of long white pearls. She strips down to the most beautiful white lingerie and keeps the pearls on to twirl around her neck. Another student loves to wear jeans, a plaid button-down shirt, and a leather jacket: she strips down

you up

to Calvin Klein low-rise jockeys and a tight, transparent muscle-man tank with no bra underneath.

Before you learn to strip, you need to figure out what you'll be stripping out of, and what clothes best express or bring out your erotic persona. As children, we often played dress-up and imagined what we might be when we grew up. I can assure you that my childhood dreams looked nothing like this:

Blood-red crushed-velvet short shorts with an oversize silver zipper up the front; black vinyl thigh-high lace-up stiletto boots; a metallic red-and-black, up-to-my-ass minidress that shimmers like water; a black lace push-up bra; a red G-string over a nude low-hipped halter G; and thigh-

high sheer red stockings. This is what I wear when I strip for my husband. It's also what I wear sometimes when I'm just dancing for myself.

This is *not* how I started. I started with (get this!) feather-trimmed Lucite platforms, a fluffy pink baby-doll nightie, white ruffled stripper shorts, and a white hello-are there-any-breasts-in-there bra from my closet. Quite a different picture, wouldn't you say? I'm a warm, friendly

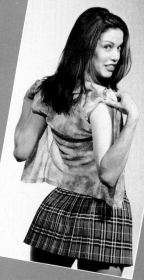

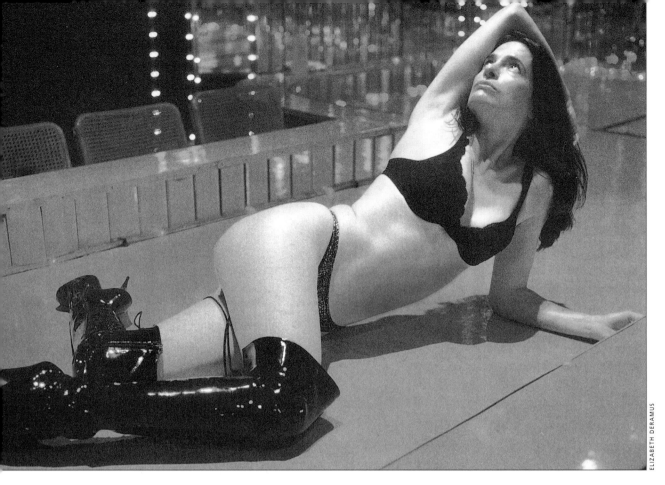

person. So when I began stripping, I just assumed that my erotic creature would be sweet and friendly. Did I get *that* wrong! After much trial and error, I gradually shed that sweet, pink-on-white image. Good-bye, powder puff. Hello, hard-ass.

In many ways, my inner sensual self was just the opposite of who I thought I was. But that first outfit, though ultimately not me, turned out to be as good a starting point as any—and I learned a lot about clothes and the way they look on my body in the process.

We're going to begin playing with clothes—trying on different personas by trying on different outfits in an attempt to arrive at your true erotic self. But before we get started, let's be frank: Nobody looks good in everything. Why do you think they invented dressing rooms? Even women whose bodies you think are "perfect" need to try clothes on, and those women discard a good 80 percent of what they bring in with them. Every body is different, and everyone looks good (and bad) in different things. So don't get disheartened during this search. The key is to know what your strengths and weaknesses are—and how to deal with them. Before you start, do the body-image exercise on page 117.

Thigh-high stiletto boots, a red G-string, and black lace bra best express Sheila's erotic creature.

THE STRIPPER STARTER KIT

ere's the foundation upon which you can build the layers of your erotic persona's outfit. You can always come back to this basic outfit when dancing for yourself or for someone else.

The Bra. Think of a bra as a frame that displays and presents your breasts like the works of art they are. Most important, find a bra that makes your breasts look and feel voluminous. It should uplift, flatter, and, most of all, exaggerate your breast size.

Yup, I'm talking cleavage here. The best way to achieve this effect is to wear a bra that's one cup size too small. Even small breasts are amazingly accented by a too-small bra. Gossamer and Victoria's Secret both make fantastic lifting bras. And of course, there's an ever-widening variety of padded and push-up bras (they don't call them "Miracle" or "Wonder" bras for nothing). Thin straps are a must. A low, thin strap in back is good, too.

Set aside a couple of hours, go to the mall, and try them all on. Pick up every bra that even remotely appeals to you, including those you might never have considered under "normal" circumstances. Skimpy see-through bras, padded bras, push-up bras, front-closure bras, bras with bows. Go for something lacy, something corsetlike, something strapless. Try different colors. My students wear all sorts of colors: black, teal, pink, nude, silver. But the most popular color by far is red. Let your imagination and tastes run wild.

The G-String/Thong. The difference between a G-string and a thong is about one inch. A thong has a strip of fabric that runs between the legs, while a G has just a strip of elastic. The lines between the two are becoming blurred, however—there are string thongs and thong-sided G-strings. So for simplicity, I've used the term G-string in the book as

The Basics:

1. Bra
2. G-string/Thong
3. Stripper shorts
4. Top (T-shirt, dress, or tank)
5. 6-inch heels

the item of clothing worn on the bottom. The G-string or thong that you wear for stripping is not your average flimsy one. You need to get yourself a sturdy, well-constructed, professional thong or G-string—one that covers your entire vulva area even when your legs are spread.

Try on a G-string over tights or panty hose (rather than underwear) so that you can clearly see the line and tell whether a particular style flatters your leg and body type. Give each style a "test run": stand with your back to the mirror, bend down, and peer between your legs. Then sit on the floor facing the mirror, spread your legs as wide as you can, and scissor them (I'm serious). The G-string should stay in place throughout. If not, keep looking.

Here are some tips about choosing a G-string style that flatters your figure: A high cut on the hips makes the legs appear longer. A hip-hugger thong makes the waist look longer. Those looking for a bit more support should opt for the halter or thong-style G rather than the string-tie. Color-coordinating the thong with your bra makes the line of your body look longer—a plus for just about anyone.

Stripper Shorts. The word *shorts* is a vast overstatement here; imagine a pair of hot pants, only smaller. I kid you not. Stripper shorts sit low on the hip and high on the butt. They're the

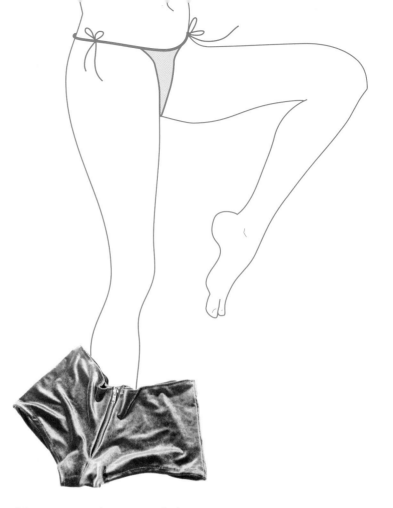

ultimate sexpot bottom, and chances are you'll be a little scared to try them at first. Trust me and take the plunge.

Your quest for stripper shorts will take you to specialty stores. If there's a shop in your town that sells corsets and G-strings, you've probably driven or walked past it thinking, "I wonder who goes in there?" Bring a girlfriend for moral support—I guarantee she'll end up trying on a few things herself. If there is no such store in your area, look online. Be sure the e-store has a return policy, since you'll need to see how the shorts look on you. If you'd rather just

Short Cuts

Here are some of the basic cuts to help you match the style to your body type:

1. High-waisted. These are best if you are long-waisted.

2. Low-waisted. If you're short-waisted, these will extend the line of the torso. If you have no hips, they give the illusion that you do.

3. High-cut on sides. These can work well on short-legged women, because they extend the line of the leg.

4. High-cut in front. These shorts extend the line of your legs and still give you some coverage in the hip area. They're also good if you've got saddlebags.

5. High-cut in back. These extend the line of your legs and also give a sexy view of the area where the butt meets the leg. Great on many, though if your butt lacks tone, they can be less than flattering.

go to a lingerie store, some companies make boy-cut panties that function very nicely as stripper shorts: Cosabella, Biatta, and Only Hearts are three I like.

Stripper shorts come in every material from lycra, lace, vinyl, and crushed velvet, and in styles like zipper-front, lace-up, and ruffle-butt. Stretch material works well for many, but don't get something too tight—too much elastic can create a bulge in the flesh around the short. As you can see, there are no rules. Try on everything, even things you think wouldn't look good on you. You might be surprised.

You'll probably want to wear a G-string under your stripper shorts, even if you don't take them off during your routine. Nothing looks sexier than pulling at the G-string above the waist of your shorts as you walk or writhe.

The Top. What you want in a top is something that looks great on and is fun to take off. You've got a lot of choices here. Button-down, sweater, a simple tank or T-shirt, a short dress or a baby-doll nightie. Buttons add suspense during your strip, but shimmying out of a tank top can be just as breathtaking. In the world of tank tops and T-shirts, there are many different cuts and styles. For example, my shoulders are wide, so T-shirts don't look as good as a halter or spaghetti straps. Does a baby tee work for you, or are you better off in a

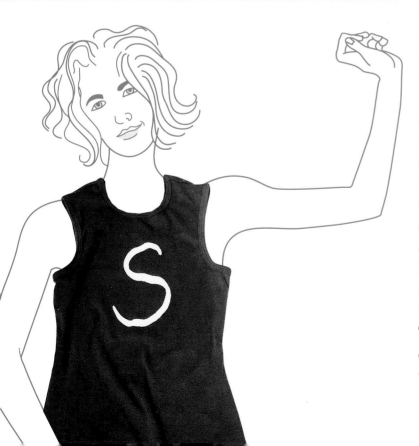

A Picture's Worth a Thousand Mirrors

Here's an old film-industry trick: get a digital or Polaroid camera and take photos of yourself in the clothes you're considering. When you look into a mirror, you first and foremost see "you." When you look at a picture, it's like seeing someone who looks like you. This allows for much greater objectivity. I can't tell you how many times I've been at a fitting and thought something looked great on me, only to discover in the Polaroid that it looked God-awful. The truth can't hurt, unless you ignore it.

boy-cut T-shirt? Use a Polaroid or digital camera (see sidebar above) to find out which style looks best on you. Does a high-necked shirt work better, or a V- or scoop neck? Now forget how you look for a second and focus on how each top makes your feel. How about an old T-shirt from your high-school theater club? Or a silk camisole? You may think these distinctions don't matter, but trust me: I've seen bodies transform and confidence blossom from a simple change of clothing.

Footwear. There's Nancy Sinatra's walkin' boots, Cinderella's glass slippers, Dorothy's ruby-red ones, Puss-in-Boots's magical boots, and, more recently, Carrie's Manolo Blahniks on *Sex and the City*. Shoes have an almost mystical significance for many of us; a special pair can say more about us than the rest of our wardrobe put together. When I'm in my black vinyl thigh-highs boots, I feel like Superwoman, able to leap tall poles in a single stride. In them, I'm over six feet tall. I feel larger than life.

Just like wearing your first stripper shorts, you may at first balk at the idea of wearing these shoes. Given the intense balance and muscle work that is required to master platform stilettos, I suggest starting your workout in bare feet. Find your balance and center first, then experiment with high heels.

In my class, heels are optional, but nearly all of my students warm up to them eventually. And there's a reason: they instantly make your legs look longer, lift your butt, arch your back, and present your body in a purely erotic way.

There are hundreds of styles and colors of sexy shoes to choose from— slingbacks, ankle boots, knee-high boots, slides, or strappy sandals. Among my students, the basic black strappy sandal is a popular "starter shoe";

(continued on page 118)

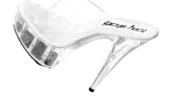

Taking a Good, Honest Look

Stand in front of a full-length mirror in bright light for five minutes. I know, I know—it's painful, but you're going to have to bite the bullet in the name of self-discovery. Look at your body with as much objectivity as you can.

In your journal, write down your favorite things about your body. Next to each, write one thing you can do to show it off. For example:

Assets	Ways to Accentuate
Good clavicles	wear tank tops or scoop-neck tops.
Nice ankles	wear capri pants; go sockless or barefoot.
Flat stomach	wear midriff-baring tops.
Beautiful feet	wear strappy, revealing sandals.
Long neck	wear hair up; or draw attention to it with jewelry.
Big round butt	wear tight bottoms that cling or a butt-skimming top.
Ample breasts	V-neck shirt or corset.
Long, lean arms	go sleeveless.
Pretty hands	give yourself a manicure, or wear fingerless lacy gloves.
Great back	wear a sheer back or backless top.

In another column, write down your least favorite things, and beside each, one thing you can do to hide or minimize it. For example:

Liabilities	Ways to Play Down
Arms too long	wear tops with three-quarter-length sleeves.
Arms too short	wear a halter top.
Thick ankles	wear boots; avoid flats.
Neck too thin	wear a turtleneck or halter-tie top.
Neck too thick	wear low, scooped necks or off-the-shoulder shirts.
Wide shoulders	wear tank tops that expose your shoulders.
Butt too big	wear a long, low-slung flowing skirt to accentuate your waist.
Ass too small	wear ruffled shorts.
Legs too short or thick	wear six-inch Lucite heels.
Boobs too small	wear a halter that plunges to your belly.
Boobs too big	wear turtleneck tops with a sports bra or bust-minimizer bra.

it looks good with just about any outfit. Another is the clear Lucite-and-plastic Cinderella sandal. Again, you won't find these shoes at Macy's. If you've found a good stripper store online or in your neighborhood, they probably sell these shoes.

When you finally do make the six-inch leap into platform stilettos, it'll take loads of practice before you feel secure in them; wobbling is a given, and balance will become a thing of the past. Keep a sense of humor about this; it takes everyone a while to acclimate to the airy new heights. Wear your stilettos around the house, on the weekend, while doing dishes or the laundry. Be especially careful on rugs because heels tend to get caught in the carpet's pile and you might take a nasty fall.

Patience is key, and it will pay off. After wearing my stripper boots for four years, I could play hopscotch in them. But it's taken that long.

Who Are You?

You now have the foundation on which to build the layers of your erotic creature. As you get to know your sensual side better, you'll find yourself going back to that stripper store—or into your closet, or to the mall, or wherever your tastes lead you—in search of new ways to express your sexuality and playfulness through clothes. Of course, there are the more common personae

The Unxpected Girly Girl: Michelle's Outfit

Michelle was one of my first students, a tough-as-nails lawyer who'd done business with some of the most powerful people in Hollywood. When it came time for her to find her erotic identity, she was sure it would be a lot like her professional personality—a ball buster who didn't take crap from anyone. But as she stripped those layers away and got to know her erotic nature a little better, away fell the black vinyl shorts and thigh-high boots she'd first worn to class. And out came the fluffiest, cutesiest, girliest little creature you could imagine. Like me, Michelle found that her erotic creature was almost the diametric opposite of her everyday self.

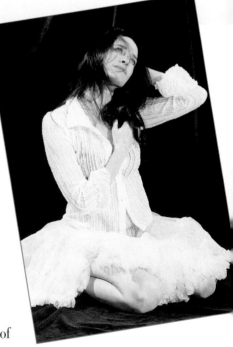

and outfits that we associate with strippers—the Schoolgirl, the Blonde Bombshell, the French Coquette, the dark exotic Stranger—but don't feel limited by them. Ask yourself: who is this creature inside you? Is she sweet or raunchy? Innocent or a hard-ass? Cocky or demure? Is she soft and cuddly or cold as steel? Or some inventive combination of attributes that's all your own?

Your S Factor practice so far should give you some clues to your erotic persona. What sort of music do you feel most drawn to when dancing?

Is it techno or Ella Fitzgerald? Which moves are your favorites? Are they the more aggressive ones, like the Wild Cat Crawl, the super-raunchy ones like the Cat Pounce, or the teasing ones like the Flirt? Look back at your journal to exercises such as "Picture This." Do you notice a common thread in what the women were wearing? Which goddess did you identify with? What sort of clothing do you imagine her in? And don't forget clues from your own closet and past—remember that Black Sabbath T-shirt from college or the angora sweater that always made you feel super-sensual. Sometimes those old sentimental or bombshell clothes are the ones that best fit our exotic personality.

Sheila in a girlie get-up (left), and her darker, bad-ass stripper outfit (right).

pubic coifing 101

Unless you're the sort of woman who genuinely prefers the wild, untended look (there's nothing wrong with that), you probably do something to get rid of unwanted body hair. I personally prefer a cleaner look. I think a hairless leg or underarm is just more beautiful. I choose not to make it a political issue; it just makes me feel more confident and desirable. And I enjoy my body more.

There are many different methods of removing unwanted body hair. Several popular procedures require a professional, including electrolysis, waxing, and laser hair removal. Of the three, I prefer laser—I've had amazing results from it. But my wallet hurts for weeks afterwards. Waxing works well for many, though there's a lot of pain involved and you have to let hair grow in a bit between waxings. Not an attractive sight! Believe it or not, shaving is the preferred method of strippers. It's quick, cheap, and it can be pain-free.

Before we go any further, let's get one thing straight. When I talk about pubic shaving, I'm not referring to just a bit around the edges. I'm talking about the whole enchilada—or nearly the whole thing. Around the labia, around the perineum and anus area, and all the way down the back of your thighs. I know, I know. It sounds extreme at first. But trust me.

1 **Pick a Shape, Any Shape.** For suggestions, see the box on the facing page. Trim the hair into an outline of the shape you want before getting in the shower.

2 **Get in the Shower.** Let your skin and hair get soft and warm before you start shaving. You may want to turn off the water as you shave.

You'll need a razor (I prefer the Gillette Mach 3), some shaving gel (it works better than cream), and a mirror.

3 **The Front.** Apply gel liberally to the area to be shaved. Pull the skin taut to create the smoothest surface possible. Many experts will tell you to shave in the direction of hair growth to prevent ingrown hairs and razor bumps. But many (including me) need to shave against the direction of hair growth to get a cleaner shave. It depends on the individual, on her hair thickness, and angle of hair growth. If you're creating a shape like the Miniature Triangle or Heart, you'll want to use a mirror to check symmetry and line.

Hairstyles: It's best to know what look you're going for before you start. Here are some possible pubic styles:

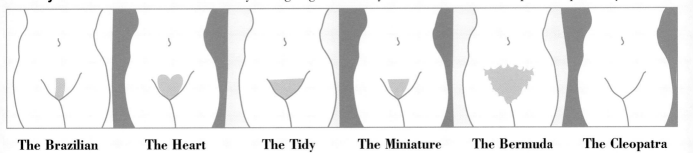

The Brazilian   **The Heart**   **The Tidy Triangle**   **The Miniature Triangle**   **The Bermuda Triangle** *(you could get lost down there)*   **The Cleopatra or Sphinx** *(shave everything)*

4 The Vulva. The next step is to shave deeper between the legs and, because you're getting into delicate territory, you'll want to sit down. If you're taking a bath, sit on the edge of the tub. If you're in the shower, bring in a plastic stool and turn the water to a trickle. Place a mirror under your butt to see what you're doing. Lift one buttock off the surface. Apply gel and, again, pull skin taut while shaving. Stroke in the direction of the vaginal opening. As you come closer in toward the labia, keep your strokes short and smooth.

5 The Perineum and Anus. Yikes! You heard right. Some are tempted to skip this region because it's hard to reach and they figure, "aw, who's gonna notice?" But don't skip this area as it may be exposed to view when you're wearing a thong or G-string. If sitting, lift your buttock even further off the surface. Again, slide the mirror under you and shave in smooth, short strokes.

If you're not using a mirror, use your other hand to feel where there's hair, then follow behind with the razor. Take it slow. As shaving becomes part of your daily routine, you'll be able to do it more quickly; but for now, take your time and move carefully.

6 Apply Skin Saver. Razor bumps and ingrown hairs are, in a word, hell. There are several lotions on the market designed to prevent these outbreaks and they work. I recommend Tend Skin, Bikini Plus, Bikini Zone, and Shaver's Choice. To avoid irritation, wait about fifteen minutes after shaving before using. Then apply very carefully to the inner regions, and avoid direct contact with mucous membranes (vagina and anus).

7 Make It a Habit. Make shaving one of those no-brainer daily activities like brushing your teeth. Always have fresh blades, shaving gel, and skin saver on hand and shave every day. A habit is a habit is a habit.

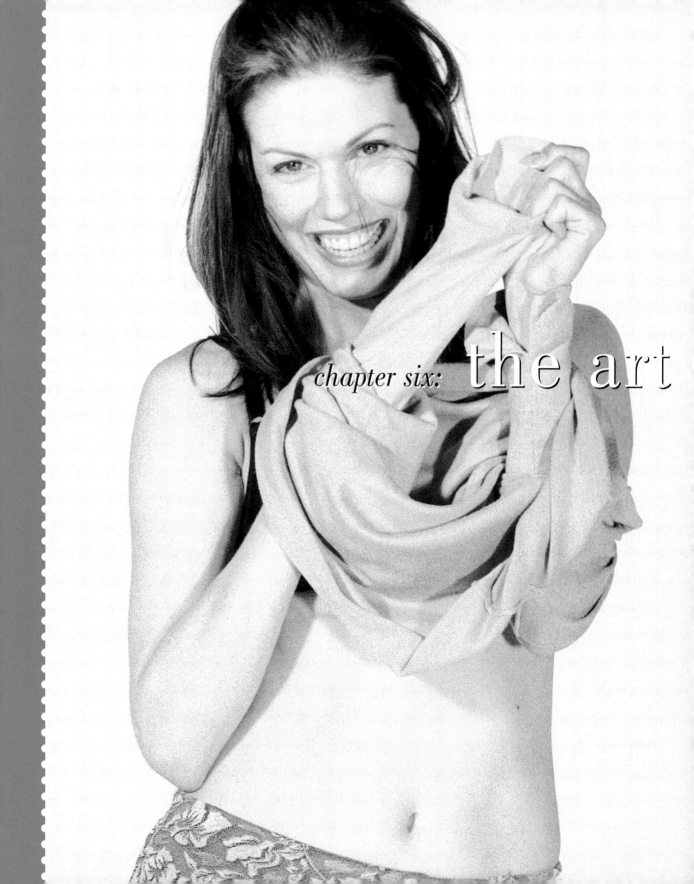

chapter six: the art

Stripping without the tease is like a Hitchcock movie without the suspense—what's the point? Teasing is all about suspense: You use your body to keep the viewer on the edge of his seat, and make his heart race in anticipation. It is the art of concealment and revelation, of controlling what gets revealed, when, and how. At the heart of the tease is a conviction that *you* (the teaser)

of the tease

have something that *he* (the teasee) wants. When you tease a dog with a bone, hiding it behind your back, holding it just out of his reach, it's the bone he wants. When you're stripping for a man (or a woman), you are the thing he wants to see, touch, devour. You dangle yourself in front of him, partially concealed and just beyond reach. Denying him your body will innocently (or not so innocently) torture him. Don't think of the "torture" as cruel or manipulative; he loves it.

He'll appreciate the gift you're revealing to him even more.

When you dance for your lover, allow yourself to go to a place that you may never have gone before. Be open to the fact that it may go beyond just a titillating ride and become a relationship-altering private moment. Let him breathe you in, engage all of you in his senses. Allow yourselves to have that perfect moment like Richard and I had, in which only the two of you exist—the place where your souls kiss.

It's important to make sure your guy is ready. Some men take a little warming up before they can see their wife or lover in such a new and powerful light. Don't push it. Let him see you in your outfit a few times; show him a couple of moves. He'll let you know when he's ready.

Although some of your attention will be focused on how these moves are affecting him, don't lose sight of your own feelings, your sensual and erotic impulses. The lap dance and strip can be even more powerful for the person performing.

Stripping

Think of the Strip as the narrative of your routine. There's a progressive buildup of the story, with each removal of a piece of clothing more dramatic than the one before.

When you perform the striptease for a lover, don't rush to take off all your clothes at once, and don't leave the whole strip until the end. Let the revelation unfold gradually like a well-told story.

Oh, he knows the clothes are coming off, just like we know that the guy's going to get the gal in the movie.

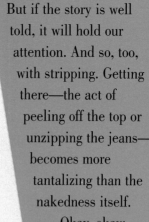

But if the story is well told, it will hold our attention. And so, too, with stripping. Getting there—the act of peeling off the top or unzipping the jeans— becomes more tantalizing than the nakedness itself. Okay, okay: it's the nakedness, too. After all, we *are* talking about men here.

Who's That Girl?

Let's face it—after years of living together, even the most loving couples start to take each other's bodies for granted. A striptease makes your familiar body new again. Instead of the access your lover usually enjoys, he has to sit back and wait for you to unveil yourself piece by piece. You've put on some music and turned the lights down; you've dressed in outrageously sexy clothes, and you're taking them off while moving in a way he's never seen before. You present each body part as a delicious surprise, a present to be unwrapped, until he can no longer stand it. You may be the woman who bore his kids or picks up the dry cleaning, but right now you're a temptress, a tease, and a goddess.

STRIPPING DO'S & DON'T'S

Do wear something that makes you feel really stunning.

Don't wear something that takes forever to take off.

Do shut off all phones, answering and fax machines, computer, television.

Do wear extra layers of clothing— the more you have to take off, the better the show.

Don't wear your support bra.

Do wear your super-sexy push-up bra.

Don't move to the beat of the song; always move to the wave. Remember, you want to evoke a strip club, not a high-school talent show.

Do exaggerate your movements—be flamboyant and flirtatious. That's what makes it a striptease and not just plain undressing.

Do arrange sleepovers for the kids.

Don't let him touch (so much more tantalizing).

Do strip to soft lighting—candles, tinted bulbs, or dim lamps will flatter your body and give a sensual glow.

Do hover during the lap dance.

Don't sit on him (too easy).

Do let your hands roam teasingly over your breasts, your hips . . . knowing these are the places his hands want to be. (It heightens your sensations and his anticipation.)

Do improvise. If you forget something, fake it. As long as you incorporate some sexy moves along with the actual removal of clothing, he'll never know.

Don't take this whole thing too seriously. Have fun, kid around, laugh.

busting out

Buttons are flirtatious and promising; they're cute and coy. Whether you're wearing a cardigan, a man's dress shirt, or a form-fitting blouse, start with only three buttons buttoned. And as always: the slower, the better.

3 When all three buttons are undone, peel the shirt open but not off. Hold his gaze and force him to struggle between meeting your eyes and his desire to look at your body.

2 Repeat the play of glances with each button as you work your way up to the top, pacing your unbuttoning to prolong his curiosity.

1 Begin in a standing or kneeling position, facing him. While circling your hips, slowly finger the bottom button. Look up and hold his gaze for a moment. Then look back down as you *slooooowly* unbutton it.

The Velcro Strip

Follow the same directions as with the button-down shirt. Or, if your erotic creature is the bodice-ripper type, tear the shirt open all at once and then return to the deliciously slow movement for the peel-off.

4 Now turn so that your back is to him, and do a slow, undulating S Walk away as you slowly peel off your shirt. Remember that your back is as sensuous and beautiful as your front.

5 Let the shirt drop to the floor as you shoot him a glance over your shoulder as if to say, "How'd you like that? Want some more?"

Wordless Conversation

When you strip, your eyes and body do the talking, so keep your eyes on him, especially when peeling off a piece of clothing. Your eyes acknowledge his presence and desire, and tease him with the promise of what's to come. Without the eyes, taking off your clothes isn't stripping—it's just undressing. Holding his gaze shows that you're aware of your own power, which is in itself a turn-on. As important as it is to hold eye contact, it's just as important to know when to look away—to give him license to let his eyes roam freely over your body.

Coyly lift your shirt to show some flesh, and ask him with your smile, "You want to see this? How badly do you want to see this?" If his response is positive, you'll know. If he seems distracted or unreadable, lean over and give him a little nibble on the neck or whisper in his ear. Wait until he's absolutely desperate to see your body before you take off a piece of clothing.

peek-a-boo pullover

The everyday gesture of pulling a shirt over your head can be quite provocative. If it's a stretchy top, you can wriggle around inside it for minutes without taking anything off. If you have long hair, leave it loose so that when you pull the top over your head, you get the unbridled effect of hair cascading down and spilling onto your shoulders. If you have short hair, it gives you a tousled, sexy, bed-head look.

3 As the shirt begins to reveal your belly and breasts, hold his gaze, not letting him look where he wants to look. Maintain eye contact until the last possible moment.

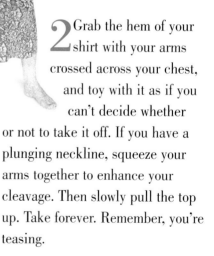

2 Grab the hem of your shirt with your arms crossed across your chest, and toy with it as if you can't decide whether or not to take it off. If you have a plunging neckline, squeeze your arms together to enhance your cleavage. Then slowly pull the top up. Take forever. Remember, you're teasing.

1 Peeling off a top can be done standing or kneeling in front of him. Keep circling your hips as you peel. (It's a little tough to coordinate at first—sort of like patting your head and rubbing your belly. But you'll get the hang of it with practice.)

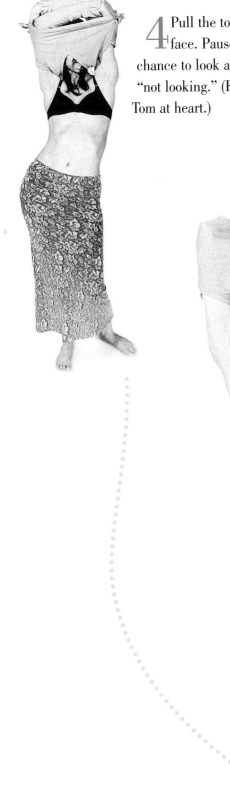

4 Pull the top inside out over your face. Pause here, giving him a chance to look at you while you're "not looking." (Everyone's a Peeping Tom at heart.)

The Three-Parka Strip

I tell all of my first-time students that, for all I care, they can come to class with three parkas on. As long as they end up taking off two of them, I'll be happy. It doesn't matter what the garment is, or which part of your body it covers—it can be a boot, a shirt, a glove. The sexy part is the act of taking it off. Keep this idea in mind, even if you're only on your second date and you're removing your cardigan.

5 Once the top is pulled over your head, gently let it slide to the floor. Or, if you're feeling especially devilish, toss it in his lap or face. "Got'cha!"

skirting
the issue

A short skirt is sassy, because as you move you can lift it and flash. A skirt is also simple to take off; you just unzip, drop, and step out. It makes a good beginner piece because it's almost impossible to get tripped up or stuck in it (although I've seen it happen).

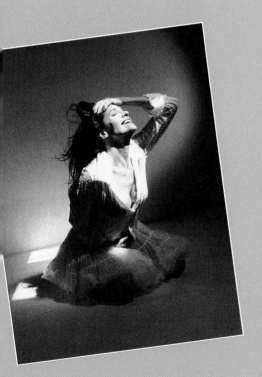

1 Stand either facing him or with your back to him. Get those hips moving in a slow, undulating S curve. Bring your hands to the button or zipper and undo it slowly, teasingly, guiding his gaze with yours. (Keep this part particularly unhurried, as the rest goes pretty quickly.)

2 Once the skirt is unbuttoned or unzipped, wiggle your hips and let it drop to the floor. (Dropping works well with an "Oops! How'd that happen?" expression, or a "Yeah, I dropped my skirt. What of it?" shrug.)

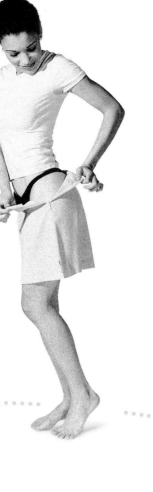

3 Step out of the skirt and saunter away. This usually goes off without a hitch, but if you're wearing heels, it's possible to get caught and trip, so be careful. (Unless your erotic persona is the ditzy, clutzy type, in which case, trip away—he'll probably find it charming.)

PLAYLIST **Tried & True & Something New**

For the strip, play music that feels unabashedly sexy to you—songs with sexual or seductive lyrics, or music with a grindy, growly quality. Here are a few recommendations:

* Marvin Gaye, *Sexual Healing:* "Inner City Blues (Make Me Wanna Holler)," "Sexual Healing"
* Bob Marley, *Legend:* "No Woman No Cry"
* Big Brother and the Holding Company, *A Walk on the Moon:* "Summertime"
* Rolling Stones, *Hot Rocks, 1964–1971:* "Sympathy for the Devil"
* Wyclef Jean, *The Carnival:* "Gone Till November"

we like short shorts

Tight shorts or a tube skirt are a little harder to get out of and somewhat more time-consuming, but remember, that's never a bad thing when it comes to stripping. The following sequence incorporates a Hip Circle, so take your time, breathe, and practice.

2 When the shorts reach your knees, go into a Mermaid so that you are sitting on the floor with your knees to the side.

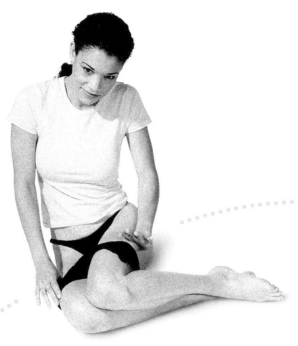

1 Begin in an upright kneeling position, and hook your thumbs over the elastic at the top of the shorts. Circle your hips as you begin to shimmy the shorts down.

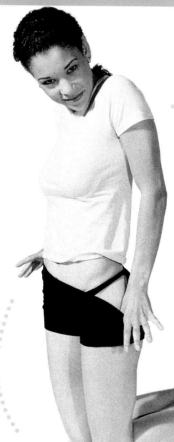

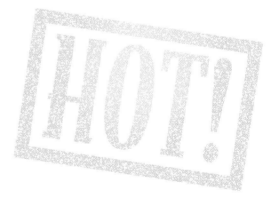

HOT!

3 Roll partially onto your back, peeling your legs up. Continue to pull the shorts down your legs. You can stop midway for a sort of bondage look, and do a couple of Fiddler moves.

4 Peel the shorts all the way off. Alternatively, you can roll into the Cat Crawl (page 92) and crawl right out of your shorts.

drop trou

The most difficult piece of clothing to remove, jeans present a challenge because the material is stiff, heavy, and inelastic. Of course, that's what makes them hot. And because many women wear jeans to do everyday errands, stripping in them gives you a bad-girl-next-door quality. Make sure you've taken your shoes off before attempting the jeans peel.

1 Start in a standing position. Unbutton or unzip your jeans with flirtatious slowness.

2 Hook your thumbs over the waistband of the pants and gyrate your hips as you peel down your jeans. Remember to take your cues from his response. If he's playing it cool, leave the jeans half-opened and go into a few wall moves (pages 98–106). Make him sweat!

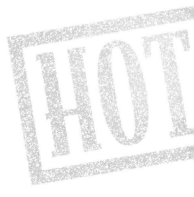

3 Bend at the waist, legs straight, and continue pushing the jeans down until they're all the way to your ankles. Remember to arch your back and stick your butt out when bending over.

4 Now the tricky part: getting out of them. Hold down the bottom of your left pants leg with your right foot as you step out with your left foot.

It's All Good

When it comes to stripping, don't worry too much about "getting it wrong." Stripping thrives on intuition, timing, and spontaneity. Focus on your own sensuality and play the game to the best of your ability. If your legs get all tangled up in your jeans, don't let it fluster you; you can do floor work with your legs stuck halfway in your jeans, and he may think it's the sexiest thing he's ever seen. I once had a student who lost one of her shoes while crawling across the floor to the lap-dance chair. After a moment of panic, she assumed this "what the hell" expression, took off the other shoe and threw it across the room, inadvertently sending it crashing through my studio window. The whole class burst out laughing. It was one of the most charming strips I'd ever seen (and the most expensive).

crowning glory

This is what he's been waiting for. It's your trump card, the ace up your sleeve—at least metaphorically speaking. By now there's been plenty of buildup, so it's crucial that you begin with your back to him.

2 Pull one bra strap off your shoulder. As the strap falls, shoot him a look over the naked shoulder: "You like that?" Then slide the other strap off.

1 Do a slow S Walk away or make gentle Hip Circles. Reach your hands around back and unhook your bra. If there's more than one hook, take your precious time.

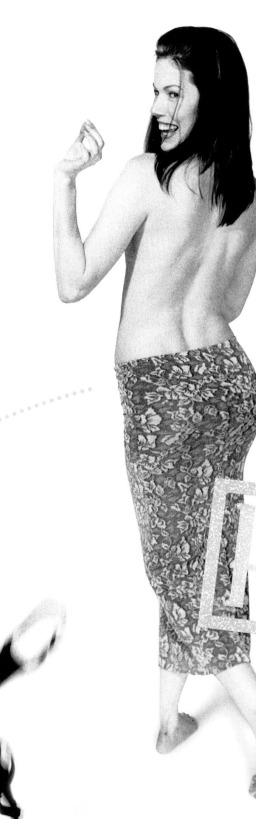

3 When you're ready, take the bra in one hand and drop it playfully on the floor behind you.

The Boy Can't Help It

A woman's body can make a man weak with desire. He can't help the reaction his body has when he sees a woman's half-naked body. As females of the species, no matter what our dress size or specific shape, we all have this allure. It's part of what we are, part of what our bodies are made to do biologically. It's not a right reserved only for movie stars or strippers; it's a gift innate to every woman on the planet. Being aware of this response and the power we have to evoke it means celebrating something we have been taught to hide or play down. Our sexuality is a uniquely female form of power, and when exercised wisely, it is a source of strength, confidence, intimacy, and pleasure.

HOTTEST!!!

4 Cover your breasts with both hands and turn and walk toward him. Slide your hands gently and slowly down, letting the palms linger over your breasts as they become exposed.

the "sleight of G"

This trick is done while wearing two G-strings and is a total crowd pleaser. The bottom G is a nude hip-hugger thong, over which you wear a tie G-string so it looks like you're wearing only the tie G.

1 While still wearing your pants or shorts, take hold of one of the side ties of your G-string and slowly undo the bow by pulling the string up until in comes undone. Then slowly undo the other side.

SIZZL

2 Holding the two front strings in your hands, start rotating your hips in large, full circles as you pull up so that the entire G-string comes out the front of your pants.

Note: It's very important to wear another thong under the side-tie one. Otherwise, ouch!

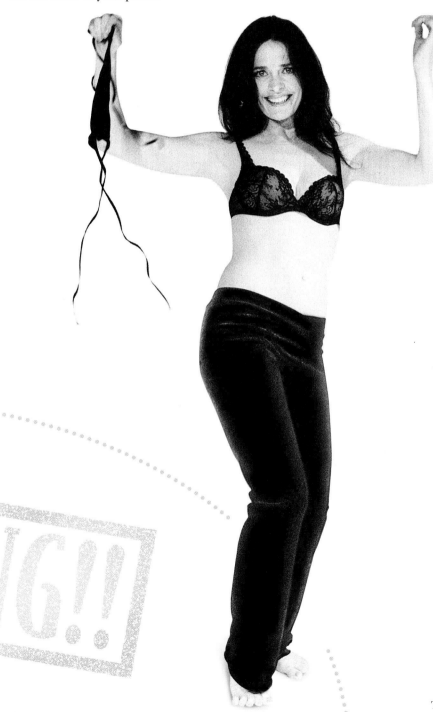

Pop the G-String

If you are stripping down all the way, you will eventually take off your thong or G-string or panties. Pull the string of the G up high on the hip and play with it. Then, keeping your fingers entwined in the strings, start to pull and tug the G down over the top of your butt and hips, inch by delicious inch. Let go ("pop" the G-string) and throw in a few Hip Circles, nice and slow. Now wiggle the G down a bit more to the middle of your rear cleavage. Stop and give him one of those "Are you with me?" looks. (He will be!) Then grab both sides and work them down below your butt in a series of grinds. Bending over, with your legs straight, back flat, slide the G all the way down to the floor. You're on your own from here.

Other Clothing

When dressing your erotic creature, don't forget there are other pieces of clothing, costumes, and accessories you can layer on top of your basic outfit that prolong the strip: scarves if you're going for the jet-set erotic babe; hats for elegance; gloves for mystery; beads and shawls for the gypsy or peasant-girl thing; sunglasses for the aristocratic Jackie-O look.

I have one student who dances in high-top sneakers and a gray hooded sweatsuit with the hood up. And out of that wrapper comes a barefoot curvaceous beauty in black silk-and-lace lingerie. She's hysterically funny and deliciously sexy all at once. Another student always wears knee-high yellow-and-orange-striped toe socks (don't ask). And when she strips down to her bra and panties, she still never lets her lower leg be exposed. You can bet that after she dances for a lover all he's going to want to see is her legs! Men! I don't claim to understand them. I just love them.

Remember, if you can put it on, you can take it off. Have fun, play, and be daring. But if something just doesn't feel like you, don't do it. You can only be who you are—not some constructed idea of what sexy is supposed to be.

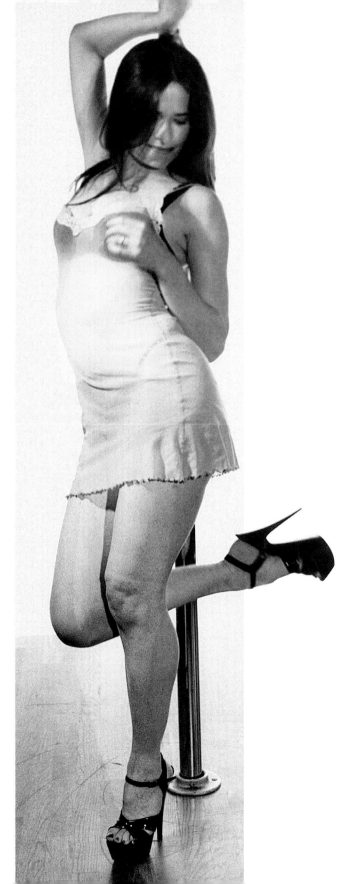

THE LAP DANCE

PLAYLIST **Touch Music**

Choose music that evokes intimacy for the Lap Dance. You may prefer quieter, more contemplative music, or a song that you and your partner have danced to (or made love to) in the past. Below is some touch music I like . . .

* Norah Jones, *Come Away With Me:* anything from this CD
* Bill Withers, *Greatest Hits:* "Lean on Me," "Ain't no Sunshine"
* Shaggy, *Lucky Day:* "Strength of a Woman"
* Massive Attack, *Mezzanine:* "Teardrop," "Angel"
* Sly and the Family Stone, *Sly and The Family Stone Anthology:* "Que Será, Que Será"

I would never do a lap dance for any man who I wasn't extremely intimate with. It's simply not a kind thing to do. Lap dancing is the ultimate tease, the portion of your strip that brings the greatest anticipation and greatest pleasure, the part that's most likely to lead to lovemaking. Unlike the rest of the movements, which can feel like a solo experience, the lap dance feels much more interactive and intimate, like you're dancing together.

That said, I lap dance to an empty chair a lot. Practicing alone allows you to get in touch with your own sexual playfulness and enhance your workout. Doing Rump Circles, for example, is one of the best exercises (aside from pole dancing) I know for strengthening your upper arms.

Think of the lap dance as the promise of a full body-on-body massage with your clothes on. You'll be hovering just above his body at all times (except in the Body Slide). If you want more contact, you can have it, but the most intoxicating approach is to float over his body, surrounding his face with a haze of your presence—your hovering breasts, your breath, your hair—all just barely and wonderfully out of reach.

Equipment needed: an armchair, a CD player, and a willing (you've got to be kidding!) partner. Candles optional.

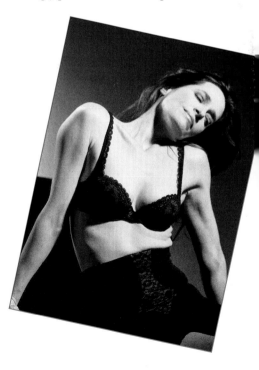

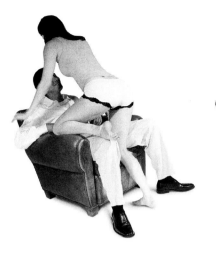

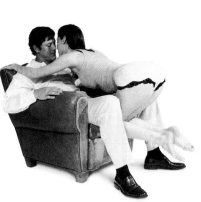

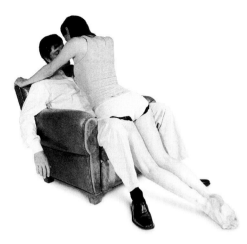

The Mount and Face Gyration

Begin by doing the S Walk or Cat Crawl over to his chair. Taking hold of the armrests, place your right knee on the chair between his knees. (If you're standing, lower your right knee into the chair.) Grab the back of the chair behind his shoulders and pull yourself up. Now place your left knee on the arm of the chair, on the other side of his right knee so that you are straddling his right knee. While holding the back of the chair, keep your back arched and draw a slow, sensual circle around his face with your breasts. Gyrate slowly and provocatively, almost but not quite touching his face.

Just-Miss Kiss and Nuzzle

The Just-Miss Kiss anticipates the excitement of a kiss, but not the satisfaction. Look longingly at his mouth as you move your face toward his. When your lips are about $1/8$ inch from his, veer off to the side and give him a nuzzle with the top of your head. Nuzzle against his neck, brushing your hair and skin against the side of his face, his ear, his shoulder.

Front Body Slide

From a mounted position, face him with your hands on the back of the chair, swinging your legs in so that both are straight between his legs. Push your hips and body against his chest and belly. The whole point of this dismount is to slide your body tortuously down his so that he can feel your pelvis, belly, and breasts.

Then, holding your weight with your arms, release your knees and slide *slowly* down, keeping your knees slightly bent, until you reach the floor.

Guys Gone Wild

While you're driving your man wild, don't let him forget who's in control. Before you begin, take both of his hands in yours and place them carefully in his lap (a submissive posture). If he's the touchy-feely kind of guy who can't control his roaming fingers, you might need to secure his wrists with his necktie. That way you won't accidentally crush his fingers with your knees. And you've let him know that you're taking care of everything.

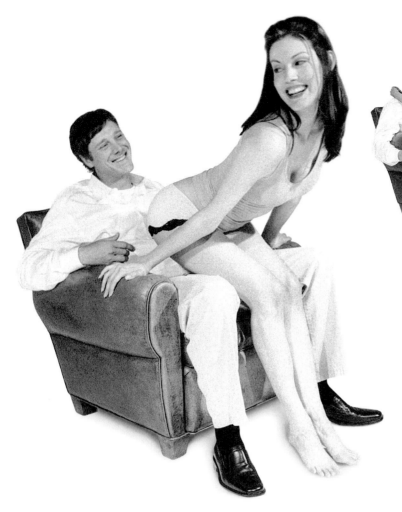

Rump Rock and Rump Circles

These two classic moves in the lap-dance repertoire are not the most subtle moves in town, but they're *very* effective. You'll see there's a reason why they're famous.

Stand in front of the chair with your back to him. Place your hands on the arms of the chair, arch your back and lower your butt so it's about a quarter of an inch or so over his lap. Your feet should still be planted on the floor.

Rump Rock: Keeping your elbows bent and your weight on your hands, rock your hips backward and forward ever so slowly so that your butt almost (oh, the agony!) grazes his crotch.

Rump Circles: Again, supporting your weight with your arms, gyrate your hips so that your butt makes broad circles over his lap.

Back Body Slide and Tush Push

The Back Body Slide is the most extended contact his body will have with yours. Sit down on his lap or between his thighs, letting your head fall back on his shoulder. With your weight completely on him, slide your back down the front of his body and between his legs, bending your knees as you come toward the floor. Scoot out your legs as your body reaches the floor and sit between his knees.

Alternately, do the Tush Push away from him, especially if he's a "butt man." Push your weight forward off the arms of the chair with back arched, leaning your torso all the way forward and parallel to the floor. Slowly straighten your legs and bring your torso upright, keeping your back arched.

RIPPLE EFFECT

Okay, now you're equipped with some pretty serious knowledge of your body's power. Even if you've only practiced alone, you've glimpsed a hidden part of yourself. Old inhibitions that had squelched your erotic power are now lying in piles on the floor around you. And you, in turn, are freer, more confident, and more yourself.

You may never dance or strip for a man; what's really important is what you know about yourself and what you're capable of expressing. Knowing how to do a lap dance should give you that same delicious sense of wickedness and daring that comes with wearing a French lace bra under your housecoat. No one need ever find out, but *you'll* somehow feel a little more irresistible, powerful, and intoxicating—now that you're in touch with your sexual allure. Knowing that you have the power to make a man weak with desire is a phenomenal feeling. One student of mine who works as an engineer among men all day gets a tremendous kick out of just knowing she could have their undivided (and riveted) attention at any moment she chose (although she doesn't act on this knowledge).

Finally, I hope you've begun to see a transformation in your body. I've watched so many of my students reclaim and reshape their bodies through the S Factor. The wonderful thing is that these changes don't come from a place of self-criticism or denial, but from the opposite. I have one student who, in sixteen weeks of taking the class, has gone from a size 18 to a size 12. She'd tried diets and exercise regimes before, but the joy and confidence she gets from the stripping workout makes her rush home from her job as a college professor to do it every day. Her weight loss is a byproduct of her journey. It's only when you truly embrace and love your body that you feel empowered enough to change it—or embrace it just as it is.

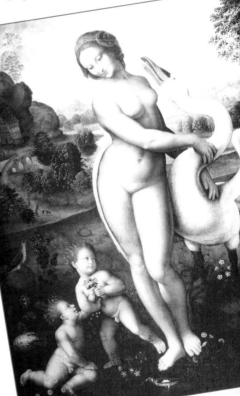

Right, Leda and the Swan, *after Leonardo da Vinci, c. 1505–1510; far right,* Two Bathers, *Renoir, 1896*

Nude Awakenings

Artists to look at:

Degas, Renoir, Gaugin, da Vinci, Manet, Rembrandt, Rodin, Modigliani, Matisse, Schiele, Cranach, Rubens, Courbet, Ingres, Cabanel, Klimt, Velázquez, Botero, Titian, and, of course, ancient Greek and Roman sculpture.

One of the many things one realizes from studying art history is how the ideals of female beauty continue to change through the ages. In this exercise, you'll look to the great painters for inspiration and revelation.

1 Take a trip to the local art museum or borrow an art book from the library. Pick three paintings or sculptures of nudes that appeal to you—it could be the pose, the facial expression, the body type, or even her environment. If you want, you can choose a clothed woman who looks sensual and appealing.

2 Buy postcards or xerox the images and put them in your journal. The next time you do your workout, bring them out. Look closely at the first painting, then roll or position your body to mirror the model's. Recreate the turn of the torso, the tilt of the head, the smile on the face, right down to the placement of each finger. Breathe into it. Allow your body to sink into this new posture. How does it feel? Natural or forced? Sexy or chaste? Like you or someone else?

3 Now roll smoothly out of this position and into the one in the second painting, then the third.

4 The next few times you work out, focus on re-creating these poses and getting into and out of them as seamlessly as possible. Soon they'll start to become your own.

5 As you begin to improvise your own routine, incorporate a few of these poses into it. You'll effectively be turning yourself into a work of art.

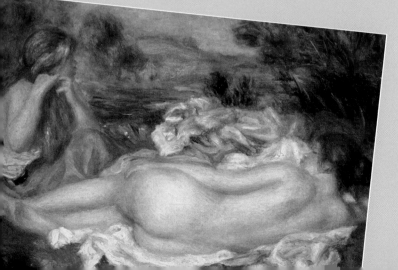

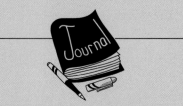

chapter seven: on the prowl:

Your goal with the S Factor (other than becoming a total sex goddess) should be to feel so comfortable in the movement that you "speak" with your body through it— fluently, without a textbook or a script. Though it may seem counterintuitive, learning a scripted routine is the first step toward reaching this goal. As with any other art, you have to master the rules before breaking them or making up new ones.

the routine

In this chapter's Routine, you'll be combining the individual moves you've learned so far into a unified, flowing whole. It's an opportunity to work on smoothing transitions so that one movement flows seamlessly into the next. Learn each part before moving on and incorporating the next. When in doubt, tackle less but focus more. I'd rather have you do fewer moves and have beautiful transitions between them than a whole routine that's stiff and static. Practice, practice, practice before doing the Routine in front of a partner; dancing for someone the first time is nerve-wracking enough without worrying about what your next move will be.

Once you've worked on polishing the transitions, begin to improvise, adding some accents (see page 160) and making the Routine your own.

The Routine that follows is broken down into four parts that unfold like acts in a drama. The first act, "Hello, It's Me!," is the phase where you let him see you for the first time. In the second, "Oh, You're Here?," you acknowledge his presence. You get a little frisky in "Let's Play." Then, in the last act, "Feeling Good All by Myself," you go back into your own world and he plays the part of voyeur again.

Begin by putting on your music (see It Music, page 149) and make sure it will last through the entire routine.

TIME: about 8 minutes

hello, it's me!

In this stage of the Routine, think of yourself as a queen, alone in your own private universe, unaware that anyone's watching. Give your viewer room here to get comfortable and ignore him during this part. This gives you the space to get involved in the music and movement. Put the music on and take a moment to just listen. Imagine the music is a warm, thick liquid being poured over your head and enveloping your body. Start moving the part of your body that feels affected by the music first—perhaps your hand, hip, or head. Keep that wave going, allowing it to spread through your body.

1 **Walk to the Wall.**
Take your time; you're not walking to get anywhere—but for the pure enjoyment of it. Focus on the soft curve of your calves as they rub against each other. When you're about two feet away from the wall, stop and put your hands up on the wall.

SEE PAGE 88

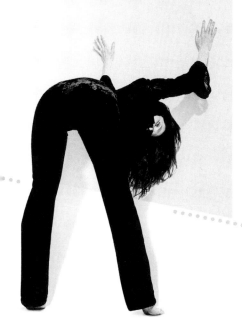

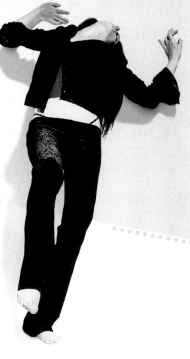

2 Frisk. Do a full, slow Hip Circle around to the right, then slowly back around to the left. Standing up, lean your body and head against the wall.

SEE PAGE 98

3 Brain Massage Turn. Roll around onto your shoulders and upper back. End up with your shoulders and head against the wall. Jut your hips way forward.

SEE PAGE 100

4 Wall Hip Circles. Make sure to push your hips as far as possible in every direction. Do a couple of slow, luxurious circles in one direction, then in the other.

SEE PAGE 102

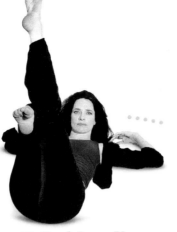

2 Scoot Out.
Put your hands on the floor, and lower your back to the floor, allowing your head to prop up against the wall.

SEE PAGE 106

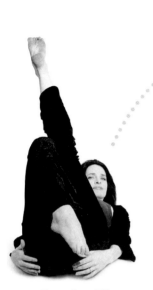

3 Peel Legs Up.
As you extend one leg at a time toward the ceiling, your butt and the backs of your legs should be facing your viewer.

SEE PAGE 44

4 Do the Flirt.
Do a clockwise semicircle with your leg, first on one side, then the other.

SEE PAGE 50

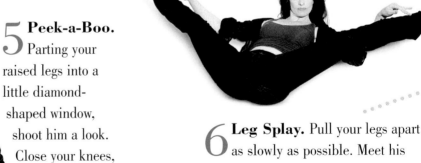

5 Peek-a-Boo.
Parting your raised legs into a little diamond-shaped window, shoot him a look. Close your knees, then do a . . .

SEE PAGE 46

6 Leg Splay.
Pull your legs apart as slowly as possible. Meet his gaze again. This moment is a dare, an invitation, and a promise. Run your hands slowly down your legs to your crotch and back out again. Slowly, close your legs and do a . . .

SEE PAGE 52

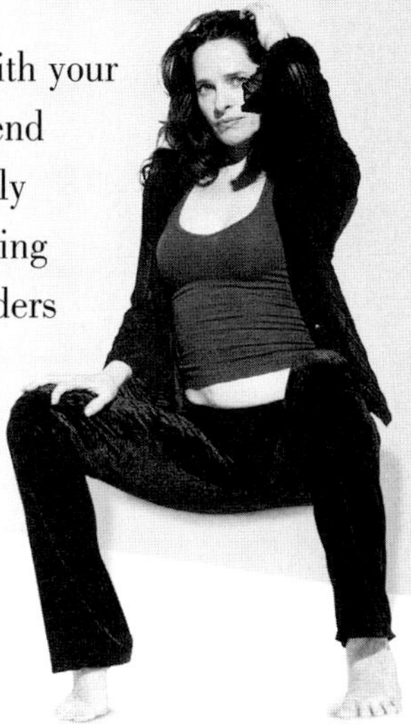

1 **Wall Slide.** Starting with your back against the wall, bend your knees and ever-so-slowly slide down to the floor, keeping your back arched and shoulders against the wall. Meet his gaze.

SEE PAGE 104

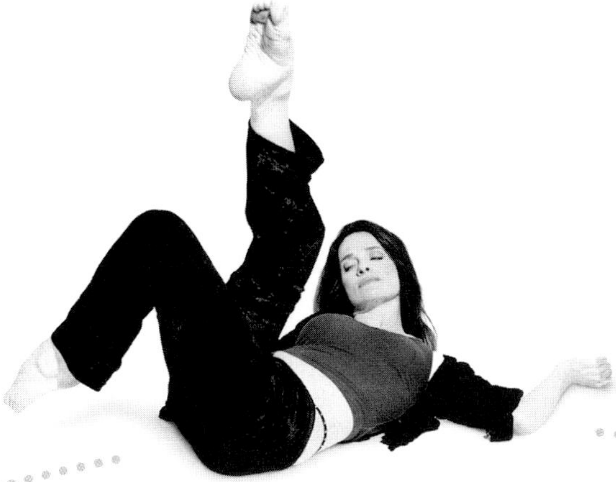

oh, you're here?

Here, you discover the voyeur in your boudoir, the intruder (though a welcome one), and your dance begins to take a more interactive bent.

7 **Crossover.** Cross one leg over the other. Take time to feel the incredible stretch in your waist and abdomen as you let your legs luxuriously pull you over onto your side. Keep both shoulders on the ground until the very last moment.

SEE PAGE 56

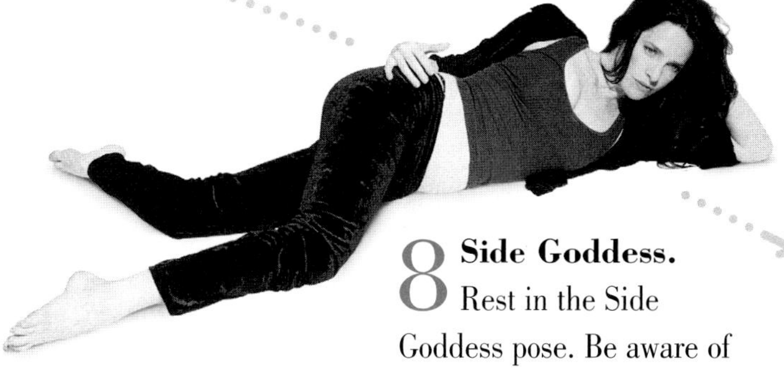

8 **Side Goddess.** Rest in the Side Goddess pose. Be aware of the beauty of your butt, hips, and waist from this angle.

SEE PAGE 56

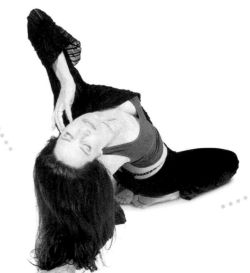

10 **Belly Roll.** Lower your leg and roll over so you are face-down on the floor. Imagine being a cat stretching in a puddle of sunlight.

SEE PAGE 61

11 **Cat Pounce.** Arch your back and slowly push your butt straight up to the ceiling as you slide your chest toward your knees. Maybe throw in a little fiery accent (see page 160).

SEE PAGE 62

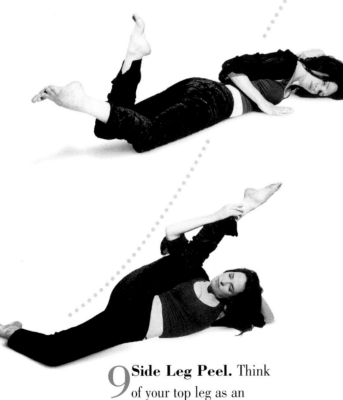

12 **Picasso Arch.** While supporting your weight on your hand, lift your butt off your feet and let your head loll gently back. Breathe into the stretch. Hold this pose as your hand travels slowly down your body.

SEE PAGE 64

9 **Side Leg Peel.** Think of your top leg as an unfurling flower in time-lapse photography as you slowly stretch it toward your shoulder. Guide his gaze with your hand as you run it down your extended leg.

SEE PAGE 58

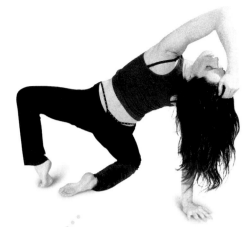

15 **Pump.** Keeping your back arched, use your left leg to push your torso up and to the right at a 45-degree angle to the floor.

SEE PAGE 68

14 **Hump.** You may do it fast or slow or any combination of the two. Shoot him a playful glance over your shoulder, "Aren't I bad?" Then bring one knee slowly and sensuously out to the side and go into the . . .

SEE PAGE 66

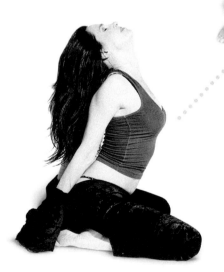

13 **Remove your shirt.** Do this leisurely. Slide each sleeve slowly down the upper arm with a warm, self-caressing gesture.

SEE PAGE 126

PART III

let's play

This is my favorite part of the Routine. It's when you finally get as close-up and personal as you want. Keep your movements slow and sensual and bask in his presence. Tune in to his scent, the sound of his breathing, the feel of his hair on your cheek as you nuzzle him.

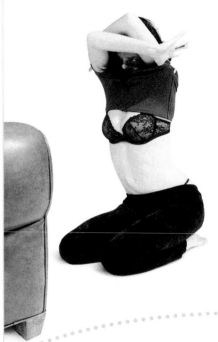

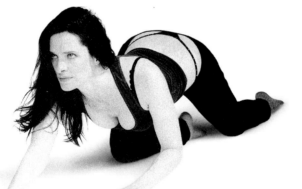

1 **Cat Crawl.** Or do the Wild Cat Crawl (depending on your mood and his response) over to his chair, stopping between his knees.

SEE PAGES 92 AND 94

2 **Peel off top.** As you do some Pelvic Circles, slowly lift the hem of your top, revealing your belly and breasts.

SEE PAGE 128

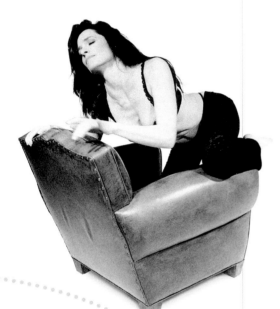

3 **Mount.** Give him a two-minute Lap Dance. You harlot of gold! End on the floor with your back to him.

SEE PAGE 142

4 **Cat Crawl** away. Let your body weight fall into each hip, giving your back a fluid undulation.

SEE PAGE 92

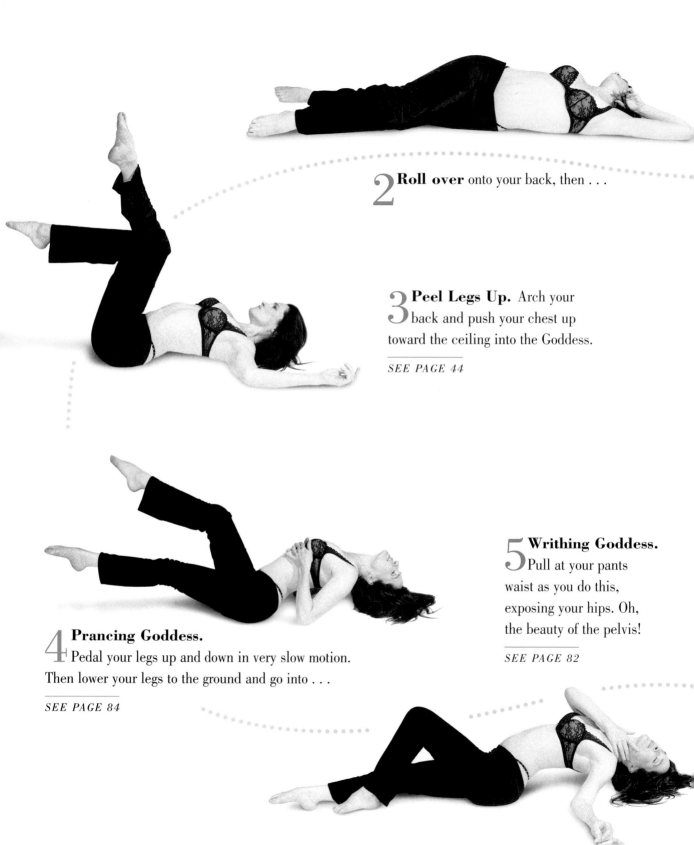

2 **Roll over** onto your back, then . . .

3 **Peel Legs Up.** Arch your back and push your chest up toward the ceiling into the Goddess.

SEE PAGE 44

5 **Writhing Goddess.** Pull at your pants waist as you do this, exposing your hips. Oh, the beauty of the pelvis!

SEE PAGE 82

4 **Prancing Goddess.** Pedal your legs up and down in very slow motion. Then lower your legs to the ground and go into . . .

SEE PAGE 84

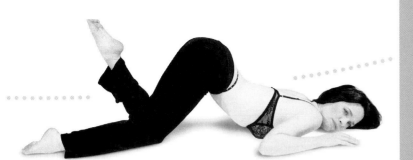

1 **Reverse Cat Pounce** so that you end up on your belly, facing away from him.

SEE PAGE 62

PART IV

feeling good all by myself

Here, you retreat into your private lair, allowing him to become a voyeur again as you enter into a state of simulated erotic ecstasy. This differs from Part I in that now you are pretending to ignore him, but he knows that you know he's there. Every now and then you can throw him a look and relish his enjoyment—which adds a delicious thrill, so make the most of it.

6 **Cross over** and go into a Belly Roll.

SEE PAGE 61

9 **Kneeling Hip Circles.** Lift one arm above the head, the other out behind you, while you continue to circle your hips.

SEE PAGE 30

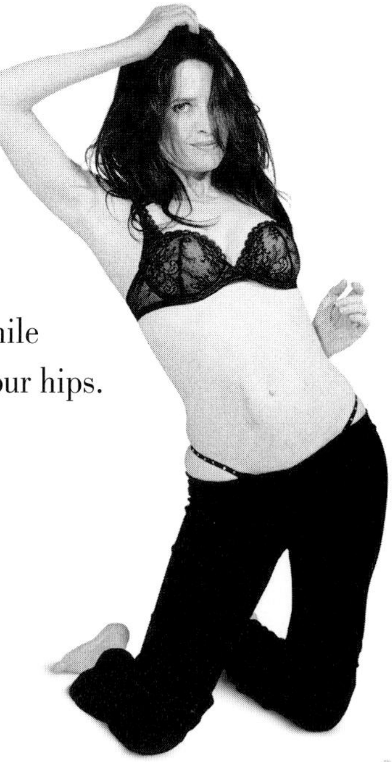

8 **Rocking Cat.** Continue the hip gyrations so that you come up in one flowing motion into . . .

SEE PAGE 28

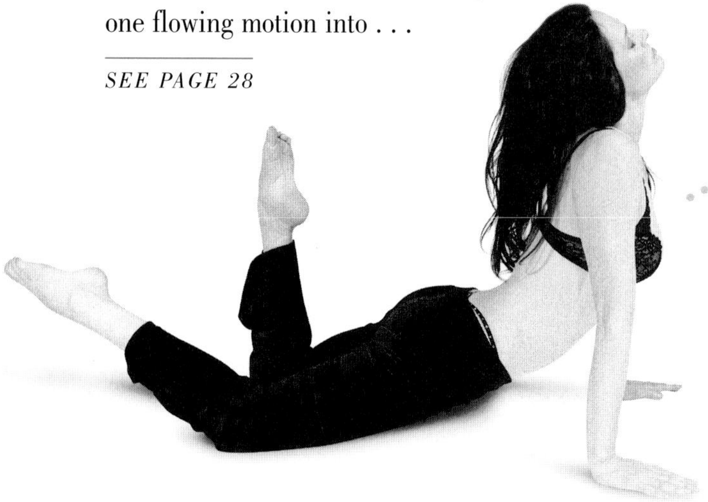

7 **Cat Pounce.** When your butt is as high in the air as it can get, go into a . . .

SEE PAGE 62

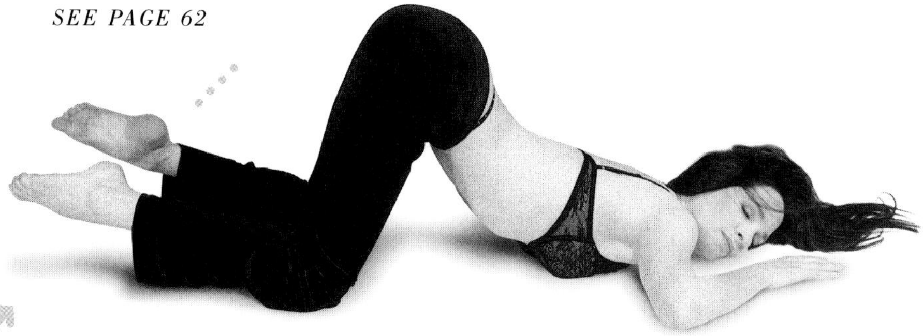

10 **Get up.**
Slowly lead with
your butt and then . . .

SEE PAGE 96

11 **Walk away.**
Unhook your
bra.

SEE PAGE 136

12 **Parting tease.** Hold
the bra coyly against
yourself as you turn around to
face him, then turn back around
and let it drop as you walk away.

SEE PAGE 137

ACCENTS

Now that you've learned the basic Routine, it is time to make it your own. We all have a mental image of a stripper who, in the midst of a slow, teasing routine, suddenly throws her head back, flinging her hair up so that it cascades down her back. That's a classic accent. (And don't we all want to look like that, at least once in our lives?)

An accent is a quick, emphatic movement thrown into the middle of all that beautifully controlled S Factor slowness. Accents are an essential part of your repertoire: they create fire, excitement, and personality, and are a great way to personalize your routine. A Hip Circle, a toss of the head, even a transition from one movement to the next can be an accent. But the quickness of the motion has power only insofar as it is book-ended by the exaggerated slowness that comes before and after.

Examples of Accents

This is by no means an exhaustive list, but it should help to get you started. Basically, these are the same moves you've already learned, only done faster. Once you've mastered the mechanics of the accent, you can throw one in whenever the spirit moves you. Think of it not as a choreographed move but as a burst of emotion and attitude.

Whip It

You may throw an accent at any point during a Standing or Kneeling Hip Circle; most of my students prefer to throw it as the head comes forward, allowing the hair (which you should wear down) to whip out in front of you as you sweep your head from one side to the other.

Begin with slow, exaggerated, clockwise Hip Circles. As your hips come around to the back, and your upper body comes forward, whip your head from left to right, then immediately slow down to your former speed and complete the

sweep. Practice the Whip It in
the opposite direction. Or throw
in a double accent, whipping
the head from left to right, then
immediately following it with a
toss in the other direction.

Hip Throw

This isolates and accents
the hip motion. In the middle
of doing slow, exaggerated
Hip Circles, throw an accent in as you
come around to the front. Whip your
hips fast around to the front and then
immediately slow your circle down to
its former speed as you come around
to the side.

Hair Waterfall

This is achieved when
the head is tossed back
quickly, allowing the hair
to fly straight up and
cascade down behind
you. A great moment for
this accent is coming up
from a Cat Pounce (see page 62).
Push all the way up so your butt is
straight up in the air, and instead
of slowly arching up into a sitting
position, flip your torso and head
straight up, letting your hair
snap back.

Wall Drop

The Wall Slide (see page 104) can
easily become an accent move with
a change of speed. Rather than doing a
super-slow, torturous slide down the wall
(as beautiful as that is), drop down all at
once into a raunchy, wide-kneed squat.

Your accents shouldn't be limited by
the examples here. Experiment with the
movements, play with the music, listen
with your body. Practice by trying to
discover the accents in a song on
the following page. You will
find previously undiscovered
accents, and those flourishes
will make the dance your own.

Finding the Accent in a Song

Pick a song you don't know very well. The point is for you to learn to pay attention with your ears and body to find where the song's accents fall. If you already know the song, you may have an idea of where those moments are; with an unfamiliar song, you need to feel your way to it. This exercise is fun to do with a friend or friends. You may be surprised to find that you all feel out the same accent moments in the music.

✳ Put on a song you're not familiar with (perhaps one of the songs in the Playlist, right).

✳ Make large, slow, Standing or Kneeling Hip Circles. Close your eyes. Focus on the music and let it move your body in ever-widening circles. Allow your entire upper body to be moved by the undulation of your hips.

✳ As you move, notice a sense of building toward something—an arc, a crescendo, even a pause. Listen with your body. You should feel your body's energy corresponding with the momentum of the music, moving you toward the moment when you will add an accent.

✳ At the moment you feel prompted by the music, throw in an accent. Remember to return immediately to a slow pace. Continue through the song, feeling for further accent moments.

throb music

Music for practicing accents should have a strong beat with a thumping bass and definitive drumbeat. For this, I like to use hip-hop or hard rock.

✳ **Nelly,** *Nellyville:* "Air Force One"

✳ **Led Zeppelin,** *Houses of the Holy:* "D'yer Mak'er"

✳ **Beastie Boys,** *Check Your Head:* "These Boots Are Made for Walking," "Pass the Mic"

✳ **Tricky,** *Pre-Millennium Tension:* "Bad Dreams," "Christiansands"

✳ **The Blind Boys of Alabama,** *Spirit of the Century:* "No More," "Give a Man a Home"

RIPPLE EFFECT

Once you've mastered the basic Routine, at some point you'll have the urge to move beyond it, to throw away the script and improvise here and there. That's when you know your erotic creature is really taking the reins. For some students, reaching this point takes weeks; for others, months and months. Don't rush yourself: you're on your own timetable.

That said, I noticed something unusual occurring at a certain point in my advanced classes. One after another, students were coming out of their routines looking frustrated and chomping at the bit for more. At first I was concerned; then, I realized it was because they had reached a plateau in their movement—they'd mastered the basic moves of a routine and were now ready to move on, to go unscripted and make the movement their own.

For the next class I encouraged them to explore and allow their instinct to lead them, letting their inner erotic natures express themselves spontaneously. Their bodies now knew the language of the S Factor. It was just a matter of letting them speak on their own. It was a turning point for them. They emerged from that next class as rejuvenated, inspired, and excited as they had been on their first day.

At this stage of the S Factor, you may be entertaining the possibility of performing a routine for your lover (if you haven't already done so). There are few experiences that can compete with the intimacy and pleasure of dancing for someone you love. It's a mind-blowing trip.

Before you make that move, I urge you to get really comfortable with how you present your body by trying some of the tips on the following pages. They are secrets of TV and movie stars that I have picked up during my years of acting.

on the set: sheila's tips from behind the scenes

To be a totally ripped goddess, you'll want to look and feel your absolute best. You've already picked out some clothes that flatter your figure (if not, take a look back at Chapter 5), but you may still be feeling self-conscious about your body. Remember, all women—even movie stars, pop singers, and models—have flaws. They have body fat and pimples and cellulite and unwanted body hair. I swear. I've worked in Hollywood for years, and I've seen a lot of these women up close. Sure, they're beautiful. But they're not perfect. The difference between them and you? They know how to play up their assets and disguise their shortcomings. Like these women, you can learn to mask the little flaws while making the most of what you've got. Here are some tricks of the trade—about lighting, makeup, and styling—that I've learned behind the scenes on movie sets.

Lighting

I've had two children and the skin on my belly is not the tautest region of my epidermis. With the right sort of lighting, however, no one has to know. Learning how to be your own lighting designer can radically alter the way your body looks.

Low, indirect, or diffused light is the best way to airbrush out your body's flaws. Get a dimmer switch for overhead lights, or turn them off and bring in a floor lamp that you can throw a scarf over. Christmas lights also give off a nice, gentle glow— sometimes I use nothing but them.

Candles create the most sensual atmosphere, as well as great camouflage for body imperfections. The flicker of the flame imitates the liquid movement of your body and the whole experience is intoxicating.

Silhouette lighting. Backlighting, in which you position a light behind you, creates a dramatic effect—he sees only your darkened shape moving toward him. It also gives you that wonderful power: "I can see you, but you can't see me."

Colored lightbulbs. I use red and blue in the studio. I can't even begin to tell you how gently they treat your skin and how beautifully they enhance the drama of the room. Try both colors at the same time. Your body will look better than it ever has.

Tanning

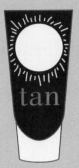

I have very pale skin, and, unlike many women I see, I'm very happy with the alabaster look; it accentuates my dark hair and looks great with my eye color. However, if you want to achieve a bronzed look, get some self-tanner. (In case you've been living in complete isolation for the past twenty years, ultraviolet rays cause cancer and wrinkles.) I recommend using a self-tanning gel, tanning towel, or a tinted lotion; in addition to giving you instant color, it helps to keep track of where you've applied it so you get even coverage. Two brands I've tried and like are Clarins Instant Self-Tanning Gel and Neutrogena Instant Bronze. The most important thing to remember before applying self-tanner is to exfoliate using a loofah or body brush. Exfoliating ensures even coverage and prevents streaks and blotches.

Body Makeup

Specially formulated foundations for the body cover blemishes and unevenness in skin tone. Body makeup comes in every imaginable shade of skin tone and is as easy to apply as lotion. My favorite is Visiora, which is available at theatrical beauty supply stores. M.A.C. also makes a good body makeup. If you're up for the investment, there's a body makeup airbrushing machine that gives the lightest no-streak coverage. The drawback to body makeup is that it can and usually will come off on your clothes, though powdering after application helps. But avoid wearing black if you use it and beware: it could rub off on his clothes or the furniture. Finally—and this is a serious consideration—you can't do pole work with body makeup on. Like lotion, it'll lubricate your skin so you can't hold the pole.

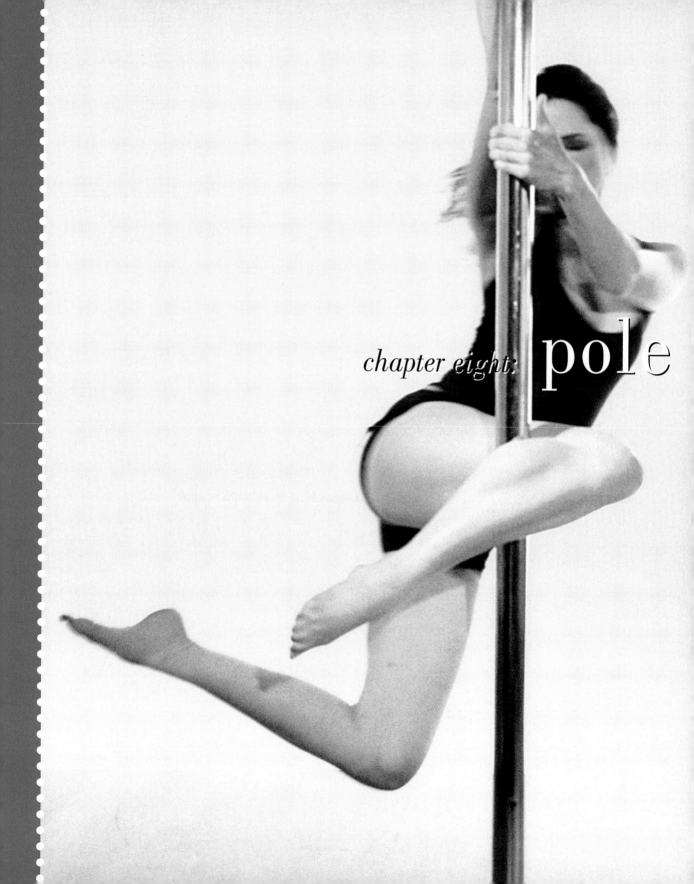

chapter eight: pole

I love my pole. If it were up to me, every woman in America would have a pole in her living room. Nothing gives you a sense of power or freedom like pole work. You feel like you're a sexual goddess, a kid, and a superhero all at once.

Because getting a pole requires commitment, nerve, and expense, I've written a lot of this book with the

dancing

assumption that you don't have one. All of my students have been driven to conquer the pole; most have installed them in their homes or offices. Once you make the leap and get a pole, you'll wonder how you ever got along without one. It becomes a dancing partner, an anchor, and a safe buoy in a sea of high-heeled imbalance. It also provides a great workout for the entire upper body.

How do you incorporate a pole into your S Factor Routine? Well, the Walk and the Wall Slide are even better executed with a pole. In fact, all of

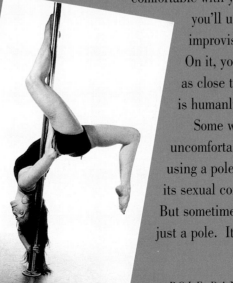

the exercises that you do against a wall—such as the Frisk, the Hip Circle, the Wall Pump—will look that much more alluring when done against the pole. And of course, there are the balletic, gorgeous pole tricks I teach in this chapter. As you become more comfortable with your pole, you'll use it as an improvisational tool. On it, you will come as close to flying as is humanly possible.

Some women are uncomfortable with using a pole because of its sexual connotations. But sometimes a pole is just a pole. It's a great piece of workout equipment for man, woman, or child—whether it's in the firehouse, on the playground, or the exercise studio. As a former ballet dancer, I think of the pole as a vertical ballet barre. It builds tremendous arm, abdominal, back, and leg strength. And it's a blast!

Always do at least fifteen minutes of an S Factor workout before pole dancing; it's important to be warmed up for these exercises.

Warm-Up Pole Work

The stretching exercises at the beginning of this chapter warm up your muscles and build strength in your arms and hands, as well as acquaint you with the pole. Do them before every pole workout to avoid pulling or straining your muscles. These exercises will also increase flexibility and strength, and after a few weeks of practice, you'll notice an increase in the number of tricks you'll be able to perform.

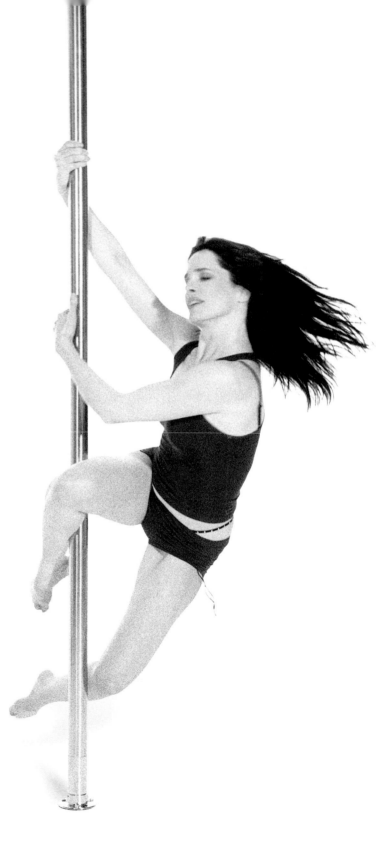

SAFETY FIRST

It's very likely that there will be a few pole tricks that will be too difficult at first, particularly if you lack arm strength. (The exercises at the beginning of this chapter should help develop those muscles.) Don't rush into things that seem too advanced, and don't despair, either. If you lack the strength for a particular exercise, you'll need patience and practice. But you will get stronger—I've seen it happen over and over. With practice, my students have gained the strength and balance to become skilled at these moves in a short period of time.

When learning a new move, take your time. To give you an idea of how to pace yourself, I teach one pole trick every two weeks in my classes. Avoid trying the more difficult moves when your muscles are already fatigued. Some of these tricks involve getting pretty high off the ground and/or going upside down or sideways.

For any tricks that are labeled "advanced" in this chapter (pages 192–210), always have someone "spot" you to avoid injury. A spotter will watch to see if you're having trouble and will catch you if you fall. It also helps if the spotter knows the moves and can correct anything you're doing wrong.

Finally, the most important thing to remember: *do not* wear lotion or body makeup when doing any pole work—it makes the pole slippery and dangerous. Inevitably, oils from your skin will build up on the pole, so keep a rag and a bottle of rubbing alcohol (for chrome) or Windex (for a painted pole) handy to wipe down the pole and your hands. If your hands are still slick and you find yourself slipping on the pole, there's a very useful product called Dry Hands available at Dryhands.com.

lean out stretches

Not only do these warm-up exercises stretch your entire body, they introduce you to holding much of your body weight on the pole with your hands.

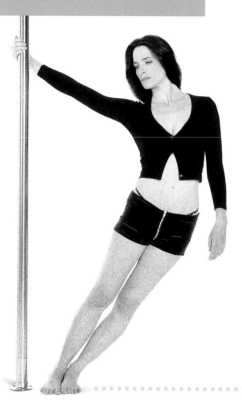

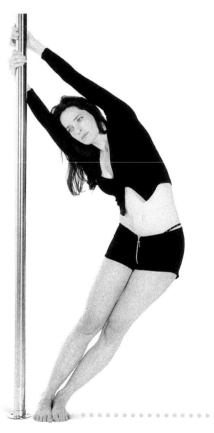

1 Stand with your side to the pole, your right hand on the pole just above shoulder level. With feet planted firmly on the floor a few inches away from the pole, let your body lean out to the left and away from the pole.

2 Stretch your left arm over your head and grasp the pole just above your right hand, staying in the bowed position. Hold it for five seconds. Repeat on the other side.

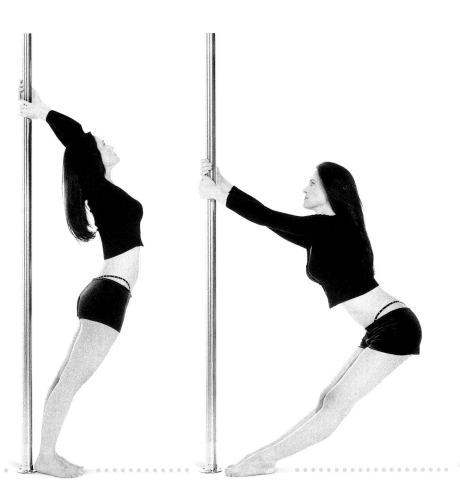

3 Stand with your back to the pole and your feet at its base. Grasp the pole high above your head with both hands. Lean your body away from the pole as far as you can. Hold for five seconds.

4 Stand facing the pole (nose to pole). Grab the pole with both hands, keeping feet planted firmly. Lean your butt away from the pole as far as you can. Hold the stretch for five seconds.

5 Keeping feet firmly planted near the base of the pole and hands on the pole, tuck your belly and push your back toward the wall behind you. Hold for five seconds.

pole hold

This warm-up strengthens the upper body, which is crucial for almost all pole tricks. Keep practicing the Pole Hold, until you've built up enough strength in your upper arms to lift your entire body. It is a prerequisite for the more difficult Pole Up (on the facing page).

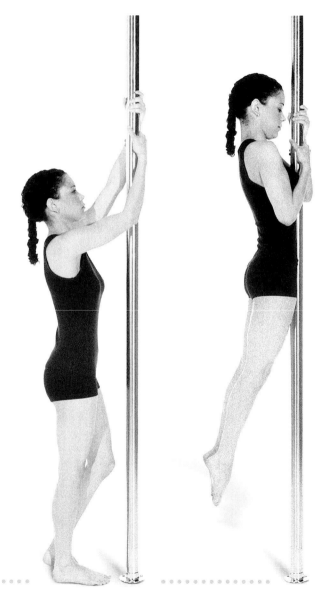

1 Stand facing pole, nose almost touching it. Grasp the pole with both hands in front of your face, left hand above right.

2 Jump up and try to hold yourself against the pole. Your hands are level with your throat or chest, and your legs just dangle. Hold this position for as long as possible.

pole up

Pole Up is a more advanced strengthening exercise. The key here is not to jump up, but to use your arms to lift yourself up. Just to give you a sense of how hard this move is, I'm able to do perhaps two on each side if I'm lucky. If you can do more, go right ahead, and may the force be with you.

1 For the Pole Up, grasp the pole with your left hand above your right. Bend your knees so you're supporting yourself with your arms.

2 Using only your arms (no jumping!), begin to pull yourself up until your face is at the level of your hands.

3 Lower yourself down slowly. Switch arms (right above left) and repeat.

swing walk

This move can be the first step in more advanced pole work or it can be a sexy move all on its own. As you walk, imagine that the pole is your dancing partner. It's something you relate to, something that gives tension and balance to your body as you move.

As you Swing Walk around the pole, take time to get a feeling for how the pole supports your body, and how it feels to suspend your weight from your hands and arms.

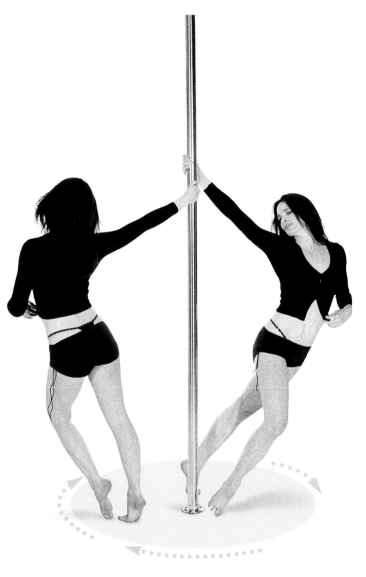

1 Standing 2 feet to the left of the pole, grasp the pole with your right hand, just above your head. Leaning your weight away from the pole, begin to walk clockwise around it.

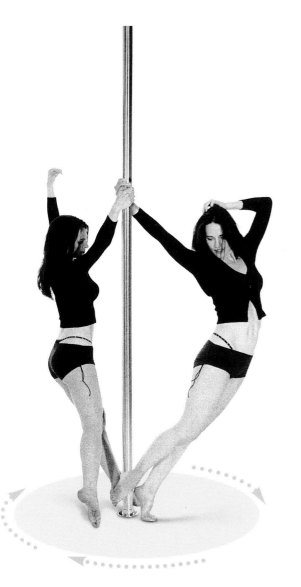

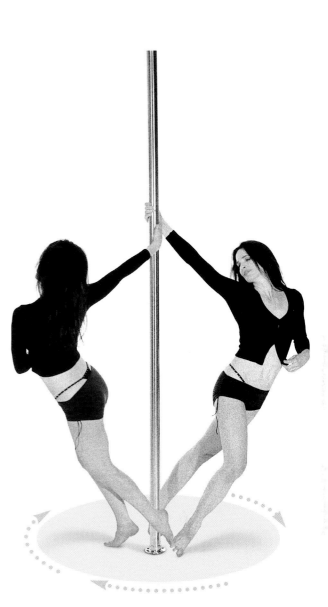

2 As you continue around the pole, incorporate the principles of the S Walk (see page 88): crossing one foot over the other, dragging your back foot through, and falling into your hip.

3 Now bring your steps in closer to the pole and let your body weight fall even farther away from the pole so that you're almost bowed. Relax with each step and allow your body to swing in a controlled arc.

Repeat in the other direction.

pole slide

This modified version of the Wall Slide looks fabulous from any perspective and is a useful transition into floor work. Incorporate it into any routine where you'd use a Wall Slide.

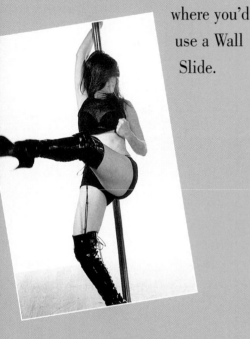

1 Stand with your back against the pole, feet about a foot away from it and anywhere from 4 inches to 2½ feet apart, depending on how modest or raunchy you want the Slide to be. Arch your back and press your butt against the pole so that the only parts of you touching the pole are your butt and upper back. Come up into a demipointe. Your hands may hold the pole above you or rest on your knees.

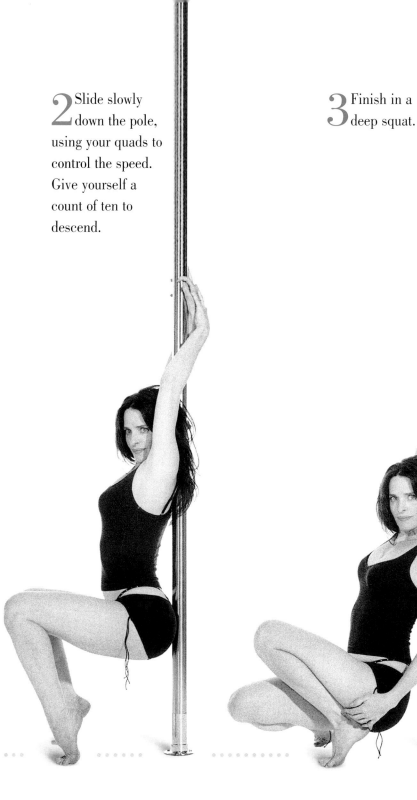

2 Slide slowly down the pole, using your quads to control the speed. Give yourself a count of ten to descend.

3 Finish in a deep squat.

What's Your Angle?

When sliding down the pole, keep in mind that you can choose to be seen from several provocative angles. Facing your viewer gives him a direct view of your face, breasts, and crotch; a side view allows him to see the beautiful curve in your back as it arches away from the pole; turning your back to him gives him a raunchy view of your buttocks with the pole wedged between them. Yowser!

pole over

This is a pole accent that can be done to great effect after a Firefly (see page 184). It's also simple and stunning on its own.

1 Stand facing the pole, with your right hand just above your head. Step forward with the left foot so it's about four inches from the pole. Press your heel to the floor.

2 Lift your right knee and hook your ankle around the back of the pole (as if you are hugging the pole to you with your right leg). Keep right foot lengthened.

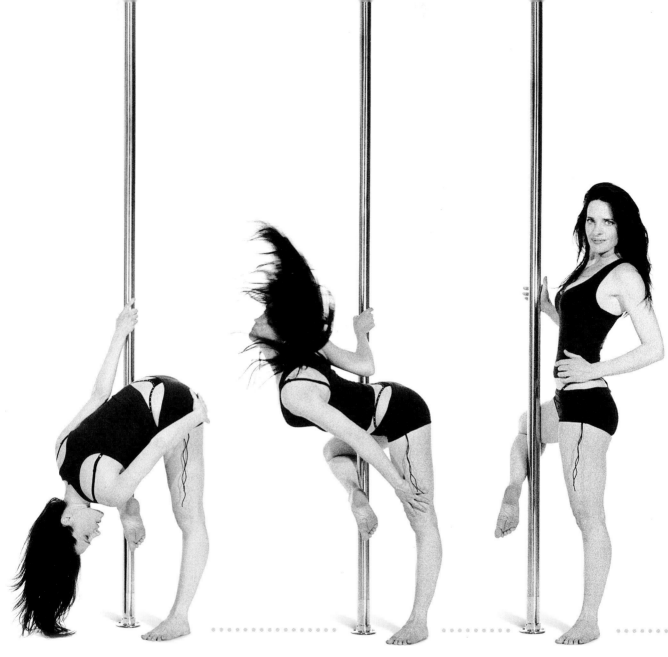

3 Bend your torso forward and toward the floor to the left of the pole. Your right hand can slide down the pole.

4 Run your left hand up your left leg slowly as you swing your torso back up into a standing position.

5 Lower your right leg.

Repeat on other side.

pole bend

This is a simple move that looks incredibly beautiful and gives a great stretch to your entire back. It's also a graceful transition to floor work. The Pole Bend requires serious muscle control—control your speed as you come down onto the floor so that each vertebra touches the floor, one by one, like individual pearls on a necklace.

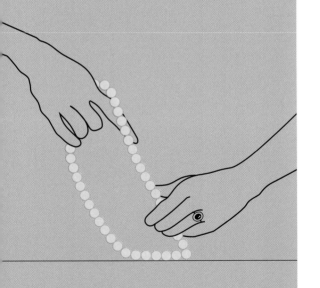

1 Stand with your back to the pole, about 1½ feet from it, slightly off center so that the pole is aligned with your right shoulder.

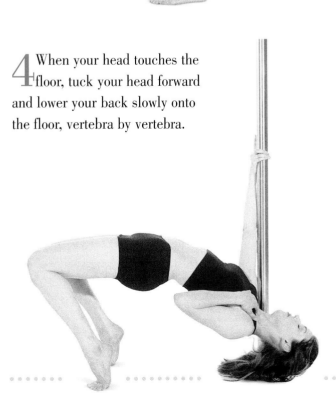

4 When your head touches the floor, tuck your head forward and lower your back slowly onto the floor, vertebra by vertebra.

2 Reach up and behind you with your right hand and wrap it around the outside of the pole. Arch your back, letting your right shoulder lean against the pole. As you drop your head down, push your hips and belly up toward the ceiling.

3 Keeping the arch in your back, come up into a demipointe with your knees bent. Then slowly lower your head down to the floor (or as close as you can get), using your right hand's grasp on the pole to control your speed downward.

5 Take your time, lowering your back one vertebra at a time. As you do this, you will be straightening out your spine along the floor.

6 Continue until your entire back is on the floor.

Repeat on other side.

pole spin

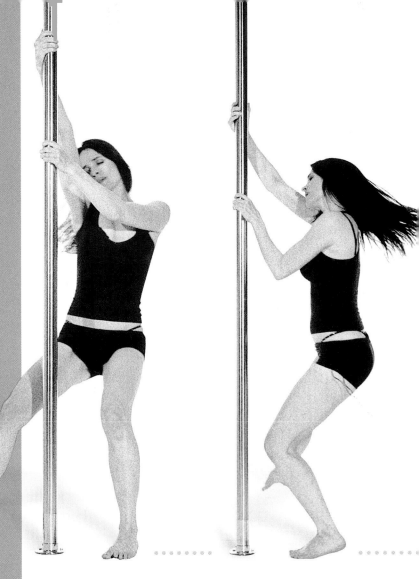

This move is not physically demanding, although the logistics are tough to master at first. Once your body gets a feel for it, however, it's like riding a bike: you don't forget. It helps to think of the pole as your dancing partner here, spinning you around under your own right arm.

Although I've broken the motion down into steps, it's important that each one flows directly into the next so that you maintain momentum for the pivot.

1 Stand facing the pole with your feet a little more than shoulder-width apart. Grasp the pole above your head with both hands, right hand above the left.

2 Push off with your right foot, pivoting in a clockwise direction.

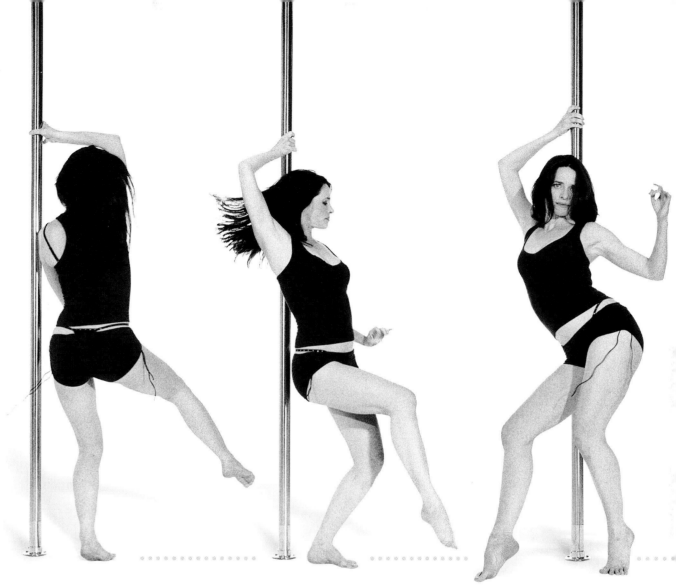

3 As you rotate on your left foot, let go with your left hand and spin under your right arm.

4 Stop pivoting when your back is to the pole.

5 Push your left hip out to the left to stop the spin. Your body should assume an S shape here, with your upper back against the pole, your left hip jutting out, and your right hand on the pole above your head.

Repeat in other direction.

firefly

Even though the Firefly is among the easier moves to master, it looks damned impressive. I usually teach it in my first class so students can feel the thrill of being airborne. Although upper body strength is important here, an understanding of the physics of the Firefly will help get you spinning (see below).

The Physics of Pole Spinning

The flying and spinning pole tricks work on the principle of centripetal force. Think of your body as a tetherball, with your arms being the rope. The rope and gravity keep the tetherball from flying out into the room; what keeps it from falling against the pole (or what keeps it spinning) is velocity. When you do the Firefly, you need to throw your body away from the pole (velocity) to overcome gravity.

Like the tetherball, your ability to spin is based on the scientific formula:

$$\text{centripetal force} = \frac{(\text{mass} \times \text{velocity})^2}{\text{radius}}$$

Though it might feel counterintuitive, if you throw your body weight out and away from the pole you will become airborne. The same principle holds for all the spinning tricks in this section: the Ballerina, Body Spiral, Flying Body Spiral, and Half-Pint.

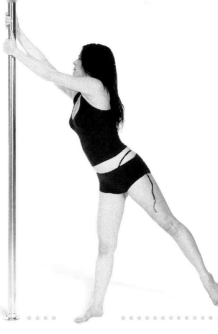

1 Pivoting on your right foot, grab the pole with your left hand just under the right.

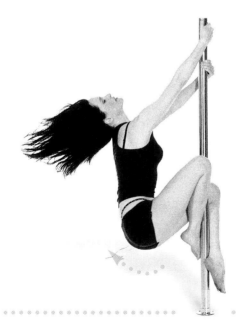

5 As you spin around the pole, scoop your belly and push out with your middle back away from the pole. Keep your arms straight.

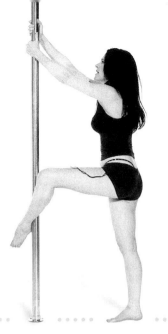

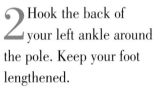

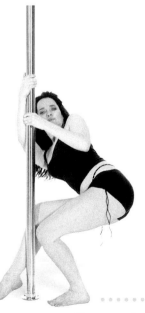

2 Hook the back of your left ankle around the pole. Keep your foot lengthened.

3 Push off hard with your right foot, setting your body in a fast clockwise motion.

4 Once you have pushed off, bend your right knee and bring the front of your right ankle up against the pole so that you are "holding" it between the back of your left ankle and the front of your right.

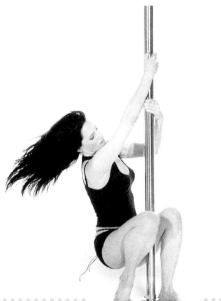

6 To come out of the spin, allow your hands and body to slide down the pole until your feet touch the floor and you are in a squat.

7 To get up, allow your left hip to continue pushing out to the left in an S-curve rotation. Slowly bring your upper body to a standing position.

Repeat on the other side.

corkscrew

The Corkscrew takes a fair amount of arm and abdominal strength. You want to curl your torso around the pole. The most important thing to keep in mind here is that just trying to get your legs up will not work; you must commit to going sideways with your whole body so that your torso is perpendicular to the floor.

The Head/Hand Theory

One of the principles behind the "muscle moves," such as the Snake or the Corkscrew, is the distribution of body weight. The closer your body is to the pole, the better leverage you'll have and the longer you'll be able to hold the trick. Your head weighs about ten pounds, so bring your head in close to the center of the pole when throwing a muscle move. If your head is up, you'll be lifting an extra ten pounds.

1 Stand to the left of the pole so that it is aligned with your right shoulder. Grab the pole at about hip level with your right hand, with the palm facing out and the fingers pointed toward the floor. With your left hand, grasp the pole in a natural hold just above your head. Step forward with your right foot, placing it between your left foot and the pole.

4 With your arms, draw your body up and in toward the pole as you curl sideways around it, bending your knees and crossing your ankles.

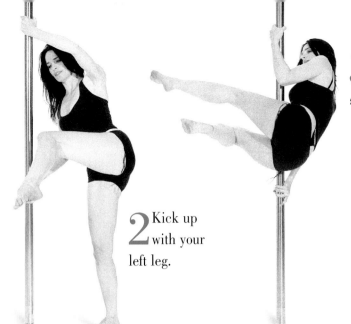

3 With your right knee following the left, pull your body sideways so that it's parallel to the floor.

2 Kick up with your left leg.

To Whirl the Corkscrew:

Use a harder kick of your left leg in step 2 and tuck your body tighter if you want to spin around the pole.

5 To make supporting your weight easier, keep your body as close to the pole as possible. Imagine that your body is a fist grabbing the pole.

6 Look down at the floor as you allow your body to slide down the pole.

7 To dismount: slide all the way down so that you are on your knees, or continue down until you are lying on your side, curled around the pole.

Repeat on other side.

ballerina

Think of this move as a pole-centric pirouette. You can spin backward around the pole as well if, in step 4, you push your body in a counterclockwise direction.

1 Stand to the left of the pole and grab it with your right hand, just above your head. Hook your right knee around the pole (so the pole is in the crook of the knee).

3 Immediately after pushing off, bend the left knee in toward your body below you so that both feet are off the floor.

4 As you spin, stick your butt out and arch your back.

2 With your left leg, push your body out and into a clockwise spin around the pole, grasping the pole with your left hand below your right.

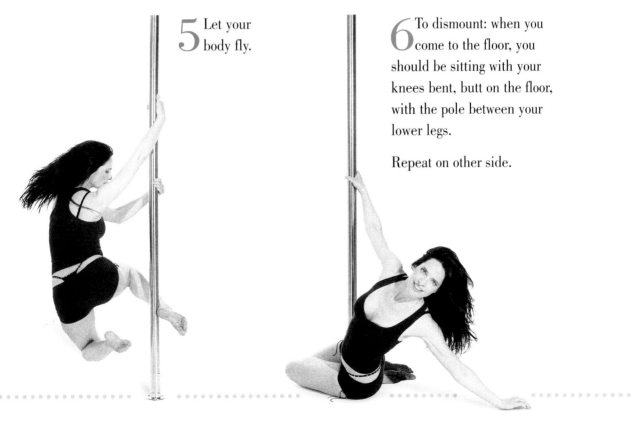

5 Let your body fly.

6 To dismount: when you come to the floor, you should be sitting with your knees bent, butt on the floor, with the pole between your lower legs.

Repeat on other side.

half-pint

Here's a very simple move that at first confounds many of my students. So study the pictures, then turn your brain off and let your body take over. You'll be Half-Pinting in no time.

1 Stand facing the pole. Grasp it with both hands, left hand in front of your chest, right hand above your head.

4 As your body spins, catch the pole with the crook of your left knee.

5 Bend your right knee and lift your left foot off the floor, allowing your body to spin clockwise around the pole.

2 Step in toward the pole with your left foot, setting it down just to the left of the pole.

3 Pivot your entire body clockwise on the left foot, pushing off with the right, keeping both hands on the pole.

6 As you spin, bend your head back and arch your back. Gradually slide down to the floor.

7 Continue to spin until you come down to the floor on both knees.

ADVANCED *

snake

The Snake engages your abdominal and upper back muscles a great deal, particularly in the mounting portion, when you need to pull your body up and in toward the pole. In this move, hands and ankles help you to stop and start.

mind focus:
The important thing with the Snake is to commit to going upside down. When you kick your feet up, remember that you are not simply putting your feet up there, but you are inverting your whole body. It may help to remember how it felt as a kid to hang upside down from the jungle gym or to do a handstand.

* The Snake and the pole tricks that follow are advanced moves and should be done with extreme caution. In several of the moves, you are far above the ground and your body is inverted. They should only be attempted after learning from a qualified S Factor instructor. Never do any of them without a spotter present to watch you and catch you if you fall.

1 With the pole close to your right shoulder, grasp with both hands, left hand above right. Take a step forward with your right foot, between the pole and your left foot.

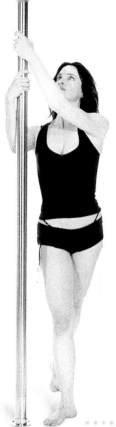

4 Using the pressure of your calves and hands to control your speed, allow your body to slide down the pole toward the floor.

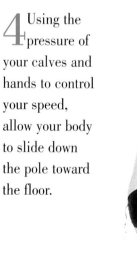

2 Kick up with your left foot and swing your body upside down as you hook the pole with your left ankle (as if you're climbing a tree).

3 Bring your right ankle up against the back of the pole so that the pole is clenched between your calves. Keep both knees slightly bent and feet lengthened.

5 When your head reaches the floor, tuck it under and let your body slowly unfurl, vertebra by vertebra, from the top of your neck to the small of your back.

6 Allow your feet to stay on the pole for as long as you can, then peel them down. End in a seated position.

Repeat on other side.

snake dive

A powerful move in its own right, the Snake Dive combines inversion and leg strength.

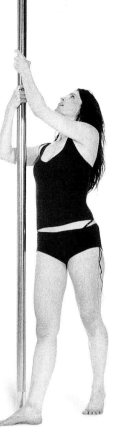

1 Stand facing the pole, with the pole close to your right shoulder. Grasp the pole with both hands, right hand at about chin height, left hand just above your head. Take a step forward with your right foot, between the pole and your left foot.

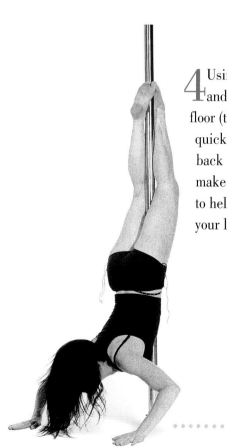

4 Using your legs as the brakes and gas, lower your body to the floor (this can be done slowly or quickly as an accent), keeping back arched. When your hands make contact with floor, use them to help lower yourself, keeping your legs clasped to the pole.

5 Walk your hands out along the floor, lowering yourself further. Arch your back so that as you come down, your torso slides out from the pole and onto the floor on your chest and then belly.

2 Kick up your left foot and swing your body upside down as you hook the pole with your left ankle. Bring your right ankle up against the back of the pole so that the pole is clenched between your calves. Keep both knees slightly bent and feet lengthened.

3 Making sure you have a firm grasp on the pole with your calves, release your hands and arch your back, looking down at the floor. Raise your hands above your head toward the floor.

6 When your torso is on the floor, release your calves' grasp on the pole. Press your feet against the pole, pushing your body all the way out along the floor. End on your hands and knees with the pole between your legs.

pole cat

A very sexy variant on the Snake, the Pole Cat was inspired by the way a cat looks when it tries to climb down a tree. (I trust you'll be more successful!)

I recommend getting comfortable with the Snake first before trying this trick. The Pole Cat uses the same muscles as the Snake—arms, legs, abs, and back—with more emphasis on the abs and back muscles. As with the Snake, be sure to use a spotter.

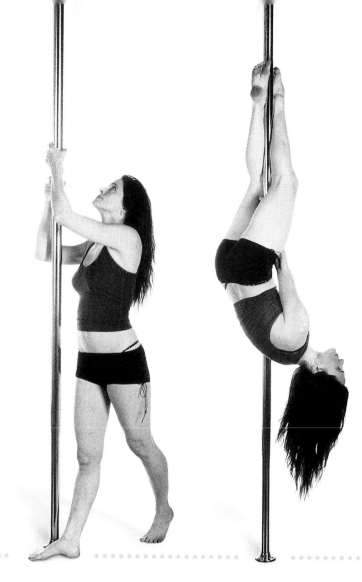

1 Stand facing the pole, left hand above right at face level.

2 Come up into a Snake.

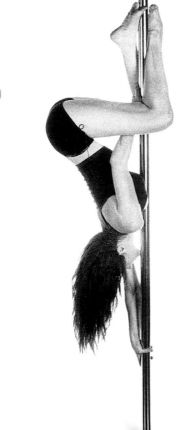
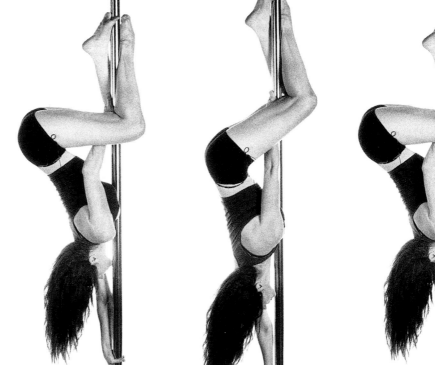
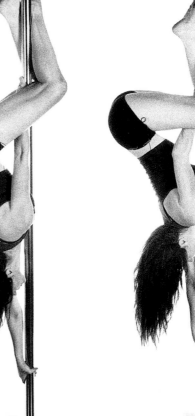

3 Extend your right hand down the pole ("above" your head) and grasp the pole with it, keeping the left hand where it is.

4 Bend your knees, arch your back, and push your butt up and toward the wall behind you, almost as if you're doing a Cat Pounce on the pole.

5 Using your arms to keep yourself secure, pump your torso down again, lowering your butt down the pole.

6 Move back up again, sticking your butt out.

To dismount: tuck your head and slide down headfirst. Uncurl your spine very slowly along the floor.

descending angel

A stunningly beautiful move that makes you looks like a member of an aerial troupe, Descending Angel requires strength and flexibility.

1 Stand facing the pole with the pole aligned with your right shoulder. Grasp the pole with both hands, right hand at about chin height, left hand above your head.

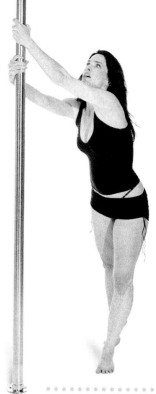

4 Hook the pole with your right knee.

5 Let go of the pole with your left hand. Arch your back and drop your left leg away from the pole and toward your head. Keep your left knee bent and left foot lengthened. Drop your head back. Grasp the pole above your head with your left hand for stability. Using your right hand and right leg to control your descent, slide down the pole toward the floor.

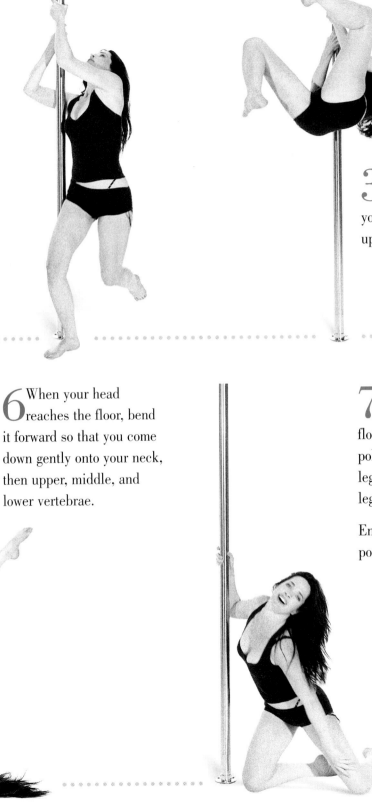

2 Take a step forward with your right foot, between the pole and your left foot.

3 Kick up with your left foot as you swing your body upside down.

6 When your head reaches the floor, bend it forward so that you come down gently onto your neck, then upper, middle, and lower vertebrae.

7 When your entire back is on the floor, unclasp the pole with the right leg and lower both legs to the floor.

End in a kneeling position.

body spiral

As with the other spinning pole tricks, the key here is to get some good distance between your body and the pole, and to get some circular force going with your body weight.

1 Facing the pole, grasp the pole with your right hand. Step forward with the right foot, bringing the right shoulder in towards the pole. Grab the pole with your left hand, just above your head.

4 Wrap your upper back around the pole. Your body should then spiral clockwise around the pole with your back to the pole.

5 Using your hands to control your speed, slide down the pole as you spin.

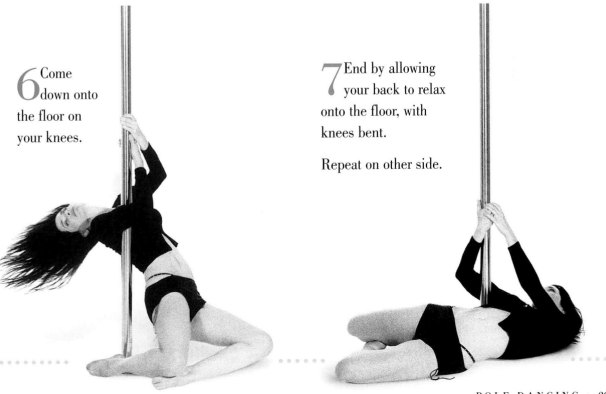

2 Tuck the pole into your right armpit as you push off with your right foot. Kick off with your left foot and swing your hips out to the left and around.

3 Keep your hips pushed up and out as you become airborne.

6 Come down onto the floor on your knees.

7 End by allowing your back to relax onto the floor, with knees bent.

Repeat on other side.

ADVANCED

flying body spiral

A lso challenging, this trick requires particular strength in the hands. Think of your entire body as a pendulum moving in a circle. I don't like to play favorites, but between you and me, the Flying Body Spiral is the most amazing move. I absolutely love it!

1 With the pole on your right side, grasp it above your head with only your right hand. Step forward with your right foot.

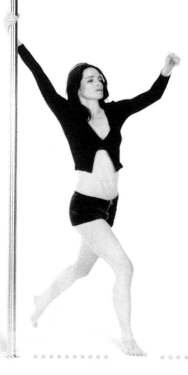

5 As you make your first rotation, reach behind your back with your left hand and let it catch hold of the pole behind you.

4 Your body should then spiral around the pole with your back to it.

2 Sweep your left leg out and around as you push off with your right foot.

3 Allow your body to spin out and around the pole clockwise, keeping your hips up.

6 Keep your hips lifted as you push your chest up toward the ceiling and bend your knees. Relax and breathe.

7 As you spiral around, your body will descend down toward the floor.

8 Continue to spin down and come to the floor on your knees.

Repeat on other side.

helicopter

The name for this move comes from the obvious resemblance of your splayed legs to the blades of a helicopter propeller. Like the Snake, the Helicopter requires you to invert your entire body and slide down head first. You need a spotter to help you, both to avoid injury and to hold the pose, which gets more difficult the longer you stay in it. You'll be using every ounce of abdominal and upper back strength to keep your body close to the pole and from coming out of the position.

Spinning Helicopter

In Step 4, swing your body around in a clockwise direction as you hoist yourself upside down. Instead of peeling your legs open, scissor them apart quickly, keeping your knees straight and feet lengthened. This should give you the momentum to go into a spin.

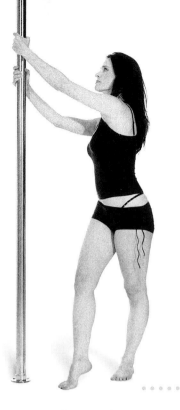

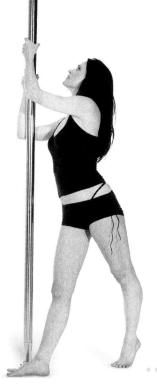

1 Stand facing the pole, with the pole aligned with your right shoulder. Grasp it with both hands at face level, left hand above the right.

2 Take a step forward with your right foot, between the pole and your left foot.

4 Using the grasp of your hands to control your speed, hold the Helicopter position as you allow your body to slide down toward the floor.

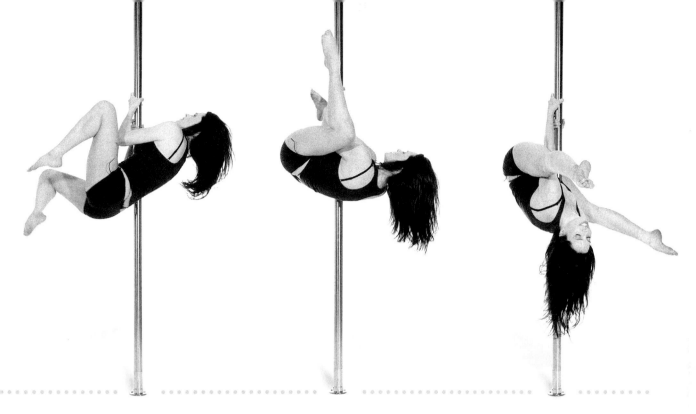

3 Kick up with your left foot and swing your body upside down as you peel open your legs, pulling your knees toward your chest, as in the Leg Splay (see page 52). You should end up upside down with your torso close to the pole, your legs straddling it, about parallel to the floor. Keep feet lengthened and legs straight.

5 When your upper back reaches the floor, slowly peel your lower back down, then your butt, and finally your legs.

6 From here, you can use the pole to help you rise or roll over into a Cat Pounce.

Repeat on other side.

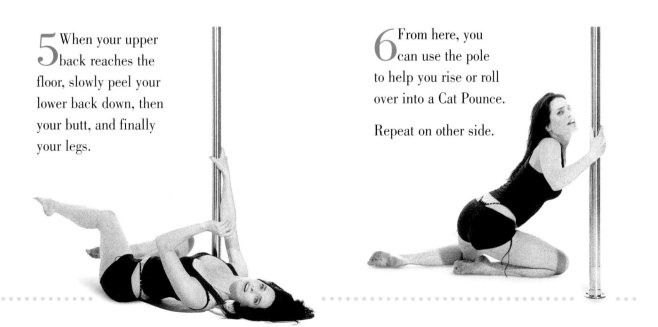

pole climb

Remember how you used to shinny up a tree or a pole when you were a kid? Remember how easy it was? Well, the Pole Climb is exactly that move, only you're hoisting a lot more weight now. The most important thing for the Climb is to learn to get a good hold on the pole with your foot. That way, you'll be using your legs as well as your arms to pull yourself up. Unless you're wearing thigh-high vinyl boots, the best way to learn this move is to do it bare-legged: your skin gets much better traction against the pole than stockings or jeans do.

1 Stand facing the pole. Grasp the pole with your right hand just above your head.

2 Flex your right foot and bend your right knee so that your foot is about level with your left knee. Hook the outside of your bent foot against the pole. The inside of your right knee should be against the right side of the pole.

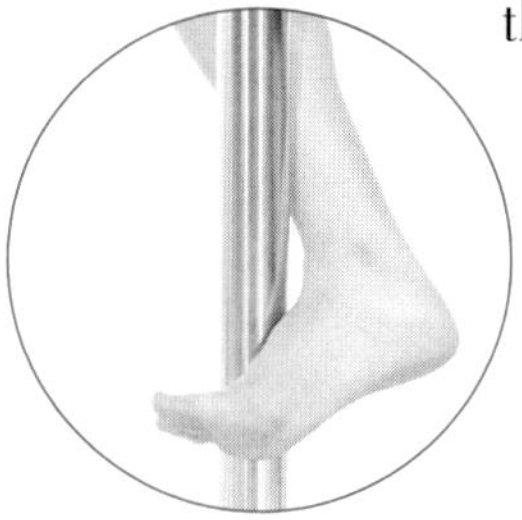

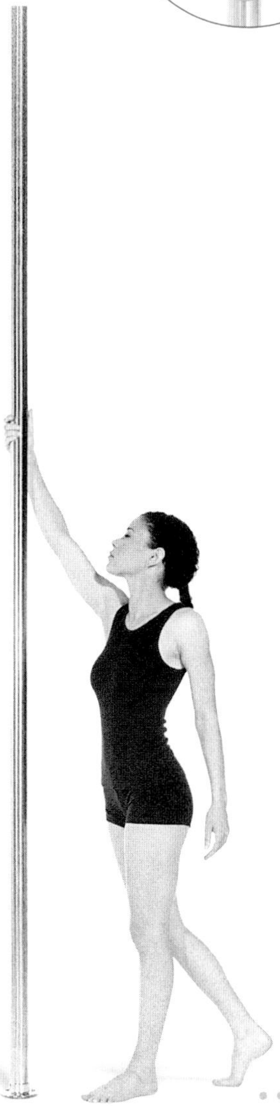

1

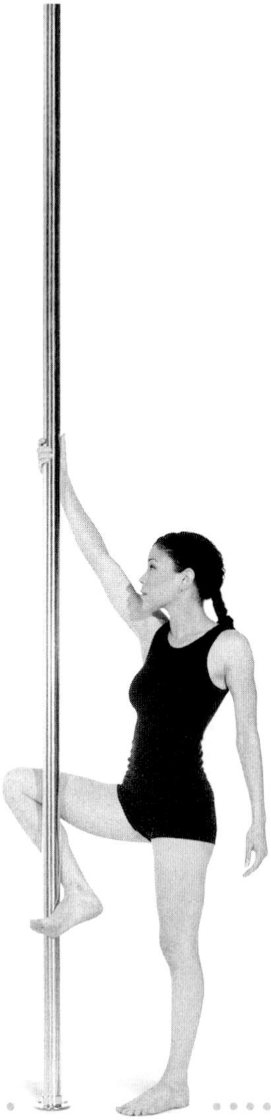

2

3 Grasp the pole with your left hand, just above the right.

4 Hitch yourself onto the pole by placing your left ankle, knee bent, on the left side of the pole. You should now be grasping the pole between your two calves and ankles.

5 Holding your weight with your legs, reach as far as you can up the pole with both hands and grasp it tightly.

6 Using both your legs and your arms, hoist your body up until your face is level with your hands.

7 Holding your weight with your hands, bend your knees and hitch your ankles up the pole. Continue climbing—arms and then legs, arms and then legs, until you reach your desired height.
To dismount: you can slide down firefighter-style, rock yourself down with your inner thighs (see page 208), or Drop and Split (see page 210).

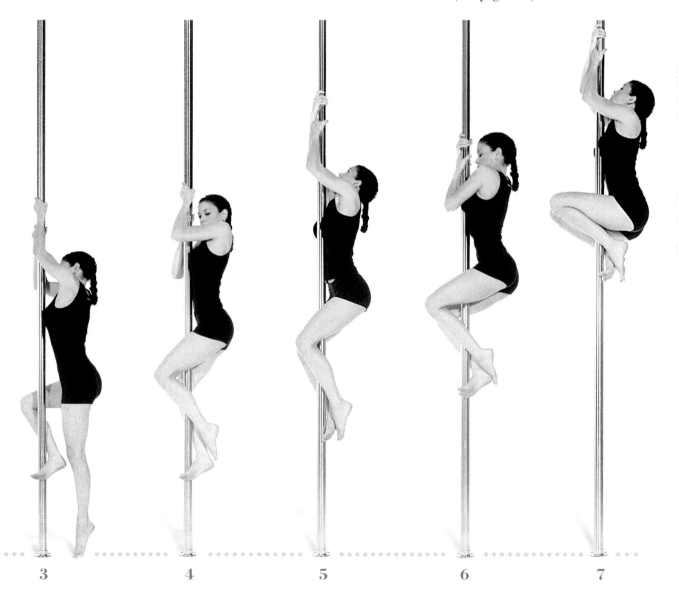

3   4   5   6   7

pole sitting

The image that always pops into my mind with the Pole Sit is the '50s one of a girl sitting in a martini glass. Some people can do this move; some can't. It's one of the few exercises that's actually easier to do when you have more flesh on your bones—that extra volume in the thigh area gives you something with which to hold on to the pole.

1 Climb the pole as in the Pole Climb (see page 206) to your desired height.

2 Keeping your thighs pressed tightly together, straighten your legs out in front of you so they are perpendicular to the pole, and are holding your weight.

It Only Hurts for a Little While

It's almost unavoidable to get some bruises when learning a new pole trick. As your body acclimates, however, the problem will diminish. Remember in volleyball how sore your hands and wrists are after the first day; but keep playing and the bruises go away. So keep at the pole work, and those bangs will be fewer and the bruises on your calves will fade. In the meantime, use homeopathic creams like arnica and Traumeel to treat them.

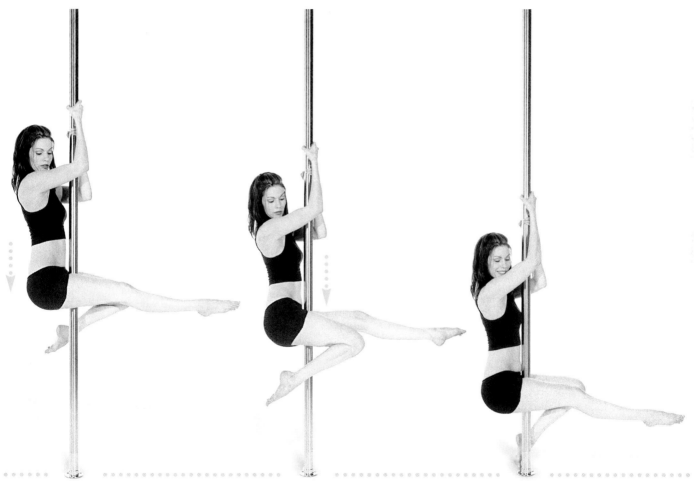

3 Prance your legs, allowing your hips to rock from side to side. Keep the arch in your lower back.

4 Using the prance to shift your weight, rock yourself down the pole with your thighs.

5 When you get close to the floor, bend your knees and come onto your feet. Or end in a squat with the pole between your knees.

drop and split

This beautiful gymnastic dismount from a Pole Climb requires, of course, that you can do a split. The Drop and Split can be done slowly, using the grasp of your hands to control your slide down, or you can drop quickly down—in which case, it becomes an accent. Either way, don't attempt it unless you know you can drop all the way down into a split.

1 To dismount from a Pole Climb, unclasp your legs and allow yourself to slide down, using your hands to control the speed. Begin to spread your legs apart.

2 As you come down closer to floor, spread legs farther and farther apart.

3 End when you're resting on the floor in a split.

RIPPLE EFFECT

Pole work is probably the most exhilarating thing I've ever experienced alone. Often after a session of pole dancing, I feel as though I've been flying. It's also incredibly rewarding to succeed at something this physically challenging. Even just learning the Firefly and becoming airborne for a couple of spins can make my students' faces light up like Christmas trees.

If you've made the leap and gotten yourself a pole, use it as an anchor, knowing that it's always out there if you're feeling wobbly on your feet or a little fatigued. And when it comes to getting a good workout, it's your best friend in the world. As you become more trusting and comfortable with your pole, you can throw in some tricks and use it to improvise new moves. Let the spirit move you.

Buying Your Pole

When shopping for a pole, it's important to decide whether you want to get a permanent or a removable pole. A permanent pole is obviously more secure, and you can climb to the top and perform more advanced tricks with it. Removable poles are convenient; you can easily slip them out of their position and store them, though you can't do as much on them and of course, they're not as safe as the ones you bolt to the floor and ceiling. To determine what height pole you need, measure flush from the floor to the ceiling. Poles that are 2 inches in diameter are the most common and work well for most dancers. However, if you have smaller hands, or just feel more comfortable with a smaller diameter, the 1½-inch pole may work better for you. Poles come in all kinds of finishes— chrome, brass, stainless steel, enamel— so choose the one you like best. Keep in mind that you should hire a professional to install your pole properly and securely. For ordering information, see Resources, page 241.

chapter nine: the shape of

I began with a story. I think I'll end with one, too. One rainy Tuesday night, a couple of months after *Dancing at the Blue Iguana* had wrapped, I found myself at Sam's, a downtrodden club in East L.A. I was there visiting Symone, who was doing double duty at Sam's and Crazy Girls. As I sat and sipped my drink, a dancer was announced: Lilith. And out she came.

things to come:
practice workouts and special strips

She stood about five foot two, had curly black hair, braces on her teeth, and was somewhat rotund. "Okay," I thought to myself when I saw her. "How's this going to work?" She reminded me of a studious baby-sitter, and not at all of a sexual goddess.

And then her music started playing—"Planet Caravan" by Black Sabbath. She began to move. And my jaw literally dropped. She moved like a floating fairy queen, all curves and grace and agility. She rolled her hips and glided her body past me as though on ice. And then she smiled over her shoulder at the audience. Her smile

dazzled. It sparked like fire. The stage lights must have hit her braces at just the right angle, because it was like a bolt of electricity through my brain saying, "Wake up, Sheila! This is the real thing!" How could I have missed it? She thought herself beautiful, felt herself sensual, and the universe followed suit. She exuded a radiance that floored me. I wanted to throw myself at her feet and beg forgiveness for ever having doubted her beauty and power. She was at that moment the very definition of sexual goddess.

What a narrow view of women and their erotic power I had had before I saw Lilith. From that night on, I realized that there is no single definition of sexual beauty; that every woman has the power to be beautiful, sensual, alluring, and surprising. It was a revelation—and since that day, I've wanted to let every woman I know in on the secret.

Expanding Your Musical Horizons

If you're anything like me, once you get into the S Factor, you'll be propelled to seek out new music to listen to and move to. Here are some ideas that have helped my students and me to keep our music compilations fresh.

* Station surf your car radio. Listen to the alternative station one day, a hip-hop station the next, then classic rock, classical, country, Latin, big band, etc. Keep paper and pencil handy to write down songs and artists that appeal to you. If you miss the name of the song, call the station— they'll have playlists.

* Amazon's built-in marketing service automatically recommends other albums you might like based on ones you've already tried. Enter the name of a favorite recording into their search option, and it will show you similar artists and albums.

* Try free Internet radio stations. Some, like Amazon, will make recommendations or "sounds like" suggestions of other Internet stations.

* Start a music club with a couple of friends (ideally, ones who are also learning the S Factor). Each member makes a mix (tape or CD) of about five or six terrific songs, with copies for everyone else. So every couple of weeks, you'll be receiving about three CDs of new music.

* Pay attention to music you like in movies and TV shows and check out the soundtracks.

THE RIVER AND THE ZONE

It's been a long time since that self-righteous 24-year-old girl edged her way into a strip club. Now instead of doing research in a dark dive or dancing on a film set, I move in a light, elegant, and airy studio, opening my chest, enjoying the flight on the pole and the feel of the clean wood against my bare feet. Later, a new class of students will arrive for their lesson. They'll be excited and a little nervous. I'll tell them what I've told you here. And we'll embark upon the journey that you are just finishing.

I practice the S Factor just about every day. It continues to surprise me, to kick my ass, to reveal parts of myself I didn't even know existed. I can't imagine a better life—to know one's body so intimately, to wake up every morning and share the secrets of that knowledge with women who want to learn.

As you practice the S Factor, you'll find that you need less and less guidance. Your movement will become natural and instinctive. Until then, you may want to vary your workout; I've included several alternate practice workouts and stripping routines at the end of this chapter to help you mix things up and keep it interesting. But as you become more proficient and comfortable, I encourage you to go unscripted. Give yourself the freedom to improvise, find new ways to link movements together, and experiment with new transitions.

Eventually, with lots of practice, you will find that the movement is a language that your body knows fluently, without needing directions or lessons. You will not have to ask yourself what the next move is; it will simply happen. I call this level of physical fluency the River, because that's what it looks like: your body becomes like water, pure movement without beginning or end, filled with unself-conscious sensuality.

Hand-in-hand with this powerful physical wisdom and instinct comes its spiritual and emotional counterpart: "the zone." You enter this state when your erotic creature becomes so completely integrated into your sense of self that there is no difference between you and her. When you find the zone, you become the most powerful, beautiful, self-possessed version of yourself imaginable. Nothing and no one will intimidate you; the confidence you feel when you are dancing will accompany you into the boardroom as well as the bedroom. Once awakened, this erotic creature within you will not disappear. She will, rather, make herself more and more a part of your everyday life.

S Factor Affirmations

Read the following list out loud.

1. Discovering my physical sensuality is the pathway to embracing my whole self.

2. Every woman has her own unique sensuality and beauty.

3. Embracing my own sensuality, I no longer need to judge other women and I will not be judged.

4. I know no body is perfect; it's only the manipulation of lighting, makeup, and airbrushing that makes it appear so.

5. I own my sexuality, my body, and my movement.

6. I appreciate how my body curves and turns in delicious ways.

7. Through the S Factor, I will luxuriate in my body's natural shape.

8. My sensuality is a good and truthful thing. I commit to discovering and nurturing it.

9. I will no longer judge myself by someone else's standard of beauty.

10. In expressing my sexuality, I channel spiritual energy.

STEP ONE

Copy the affirmations in your journal. After each, write how reading or saying it aloud makes you feel, and consider the following questions:

1. Do you identify with the affirmation?

2. Does it feel intuitively true to you? If not, why?

3. Does it make you uncomfortable? Why?

4. Are there any that you'd like to reword to fit your experience better? If so, rewrite them in your journal.

STEP TWO

Reread the affirmations as you continue to practice the S Factor. See if your feelings or attitude change. Do the affirmations seem truer, more intuitive now?

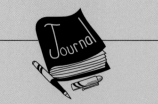

PRACTICE WORKOUTS

A workout can be beneficial even if it doesn't last for very long. The following practice exercises are designed to give you the maximum body benefit whether you have an hour or just fifteen minutes to spare. They stretch and tone your muscles, get your heart going, and keep your body open and fluid. If you practice the S Factor on a regular basis, the workouts become addictive. Soon you'll find that if you skip a few days, you'll be tense and longing for the release that comes with a few movements. All moves are cross-referenced to the original exercise.

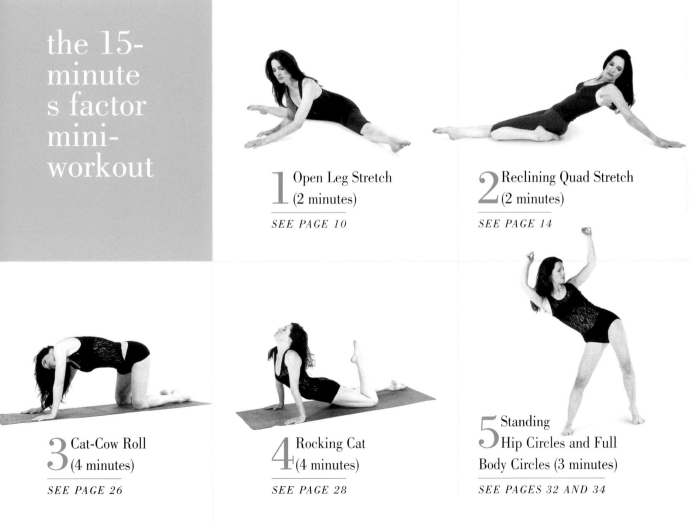

the 15-minute s factor mini-workout

1 Open Leg Stretch (2 minutes)
SEE PAGE 10

2 Reclining Quad Stretch (2 minutes)
SEE PAGE 14

3 Cat-Cow Roll (4 minutes)
SEE PAGE 26

4 Rocking Cat (4 minutes)
SEE PAGE 28

5 Standing Hip Circles and Full Body Circles (3 minutes)
SEE PAGES 32 AND 34

the 30-minute s factor workout

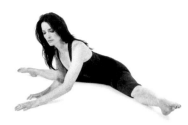

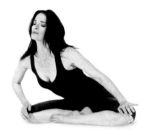

1 Open Leg Stretch (4 minutes)

SEE PAGE 10

2 Sitting Spine Circles (4 minutes)

SEE PAGE 6

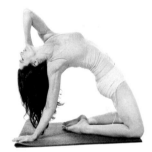

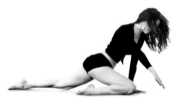

6 Picasso Arch (1 minute)

SEE PAGE 65

7 Wild Cat Crawl (1 minute)

SEE PAGE 94

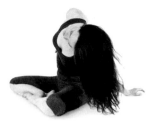

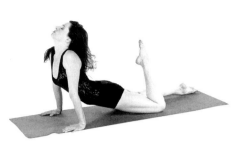

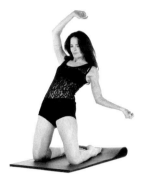

3 Inverted Spine Circles
(4 minutes)

SEE PAGE 8

4 Rocking Cat
(4 minutes)

SEE PAGE 28

5 Kneeling Hip Circles
(4 minutes)

SEE PAGE 30

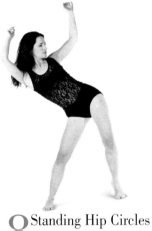

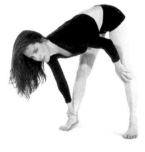

8 Standing Hip Circles
(4 minutes)

SEE PAGE 32

9 Full Body Circles
(4 minutes)

SEE PAGE 34

the 45-minute s factor workout

(transitions take about 3 minutes total)

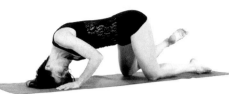

1 Brain Massage
(2 minutes)

SEE PAGE 22

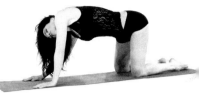

2 Cat-Cow Roll
(4 minutes)

SEE PAGE 26

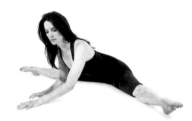

6 Open Leg Stretch
(4 minutes)

SEE PAGE 10

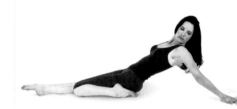

7 Reclining Quad Stretch
(3 minutes)

SEE PAGE 14

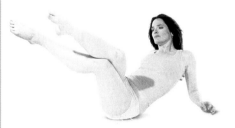

11 Crossover
(transition)

SEE PAGE 56

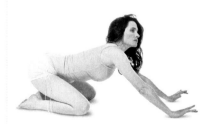

12 Cat Pounce into Pump
(2 minutes)

SEE PAGES 62 AND 68

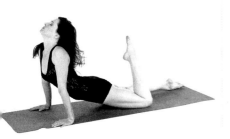

3 Rocking Cat
(4 minutes)

SEE PAGE 28

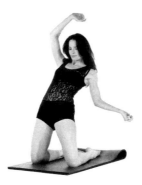

4 Kneeling Hip Circles
(4 minutes)

SEE PAGE 30

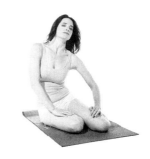

5 Mermaid
(transition)

SEE PAGE 74

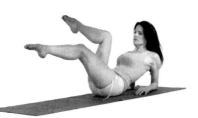

8 Peel Up
(transition)

SEE PAGE 44

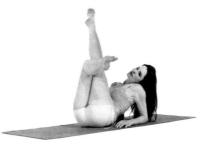

9 Flirt
(2 minutes)

SEE PAGE 50

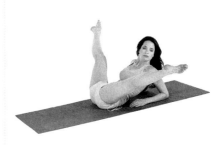

10 Leg Splay
(1 minute)

SEE PAGE 52

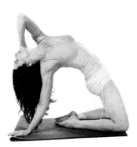

13 Picasso Arch
(1 minute)

SEE PAGE 65

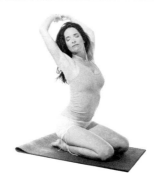

14 Slow Hump
(1 minute)

SEE PAGE 66

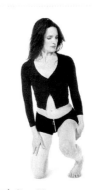

15 Get Up
(transition)

SEE PAGE 96

the 45-minute s factor workout (continued)

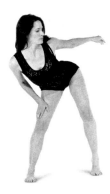

16 Standing Hip Circles
(4 minutes)

SEE PAGE 32

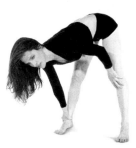

17 Full Body Circles
(2 minutes)

SEE PAGE 34

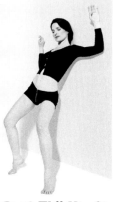

21 Wall Hip Circles
(3 minutes)

SEE PAGE 102

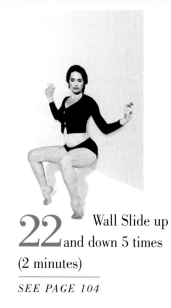

22 Wall Slide up
and down 5 times
(2 minutes)

SEE PAGE 104

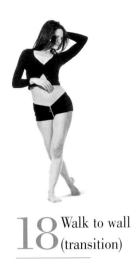

18 Walk to wall
(transition)

SEE PAGE 88

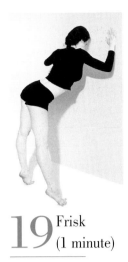

19 Frisk
(1 minute)

SEE PAGE 98

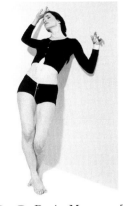

20 Brain Massage Turn
(transition)

SEE PAGE 100

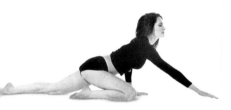

23 Wild Cat Crawl
(2 minutes)

SEE PAGE 94

s factor flow: the 60-minute advanced workout

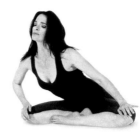

1 Sitting Spine Circles
(3 minutes)

SEE PAGE 6

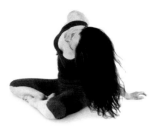

2 Inverted Spine Circles
(3 minutes)

SEE PAGE 8

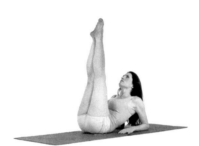

6 Peel Up
(transition)

SEE PAGE 44

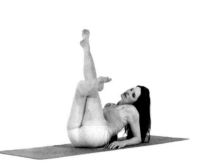

7 Flirt
(1 minute)

SEE PAGE 50

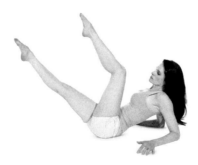

11 Prance
(1 minute)

SEE PAGE 48

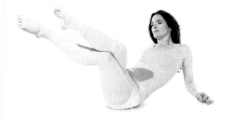

12 Crossover
(transition)

SEE PAGE 56

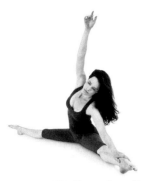

3 Open Leg Stretch
(3 minutes)

SEE PAGE 10

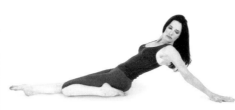

4 Reclining Quad Stretch
(3 minutes)

SEE PAGE 14

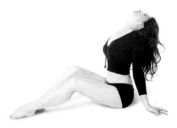

5 Goddess Rising
(transition)

SEE PAGE 86

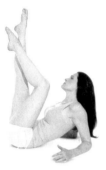

8 Fiddler
(1 minute)

SEE PAGE 46

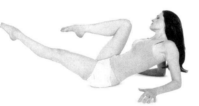

9 Prance
(1 minute)

SEE PAGE 48

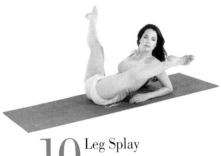

10 Leg Splay
(1 minute)

SEE PAGE 52

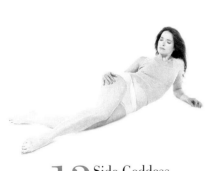

13 Side Goddess
(transition)

SEE PAGE 56

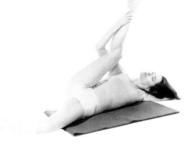

14 Side Leg Peel, right leg
(1 minute)

SEE PAGE 58

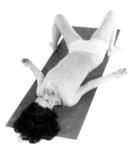

15 Bridge Grind
(2 minutes)

SEE PAGE 54

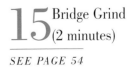

s factor
flow: the
60-minute
advanced
workout
(continued)

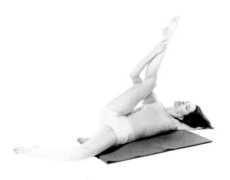

16 Side Leg Peel, left leg
(1 minute)

SEE PAGE 58

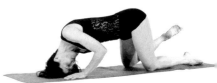

17 Belly Roll
(transition)

SEE PAGE 61

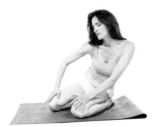

21 Pelvic Grind
(3 minutes)

SEE PAGE 72

22 Brain Massage
(2 minutes)

SEE PAGE 22

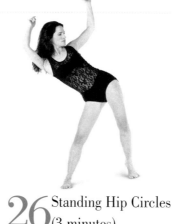

26 Standing Hip Circles
(3 minutes)

SEE PAGE 32

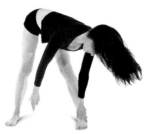

27 Full Body Circles
(3 minutes)

SEE PAGE 34

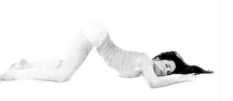

18 Cat Pounce
(1 minute)

SEE PAGE 62

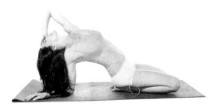

19 Picasso Arch: both sides
(2 minutes)

SEE PAGE 64

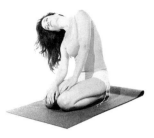

20 Sitting Body Circles
(3 minutes)

SEE PAGE 70

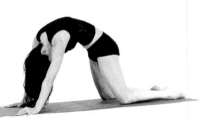

23 Cat-Cow Roll
(3 minutes)

SEE PAGE 26

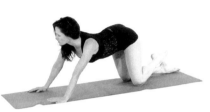

24 Rocking Cat
(3 minutes)

SEE PAGE 28

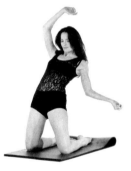

25 Kneeling Hip Circles
(3 minutes)

SEE PAGE 30

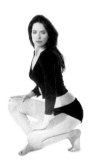

28 Get Down
(transition)

SEE PAGE 90

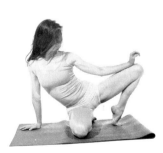

29 Pump
(2 minutes)

SEE PAGE 68

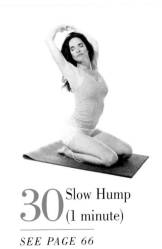

30 Slow Hump
(1 minute)

SEE PAGE 66

s factor flow: the 60-minute advanced workout (continued)

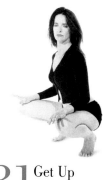

31 Get Up
(transition)

SEE PAGE 96

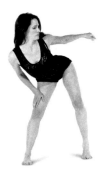

32 Standing Hip Circles
(3 minutes)

SEE PAGE 32

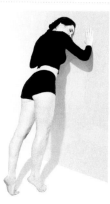

36 Brain Massage Turn
(transition)

SEE PAGE 100

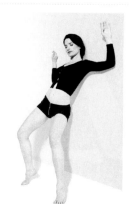

37 Wall Hip Circles
(3 minutes)

SEE PAGE 102

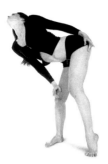

33 Full Body Circles
(3 minutes)

SEE PAGE 34

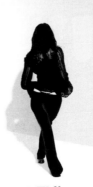

34 Walk to wall
(transition)

SEE PAGE 148

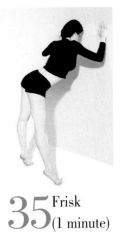

35 Frisk
(1 minute)

SEE PAGE 98

STRIPPING ROUTINES
for SPECIAL OCCASIONS

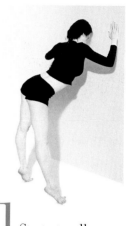

1 Start at wall

SEE PAGE 98

the quickie: the 5-minute strip

This isn't a workout—just flow seamlessly from one move to another.

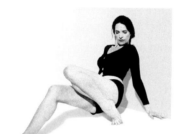

5 Scoot Out

SEE PAGE 106

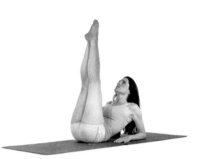

6 Peel Up

SEE PAGE 44

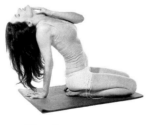

10 Picasso Arch

SEE PAGE 65

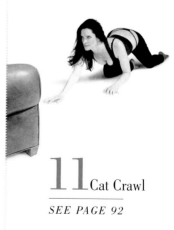

11 Cat Crawl

SEE PAGE 92

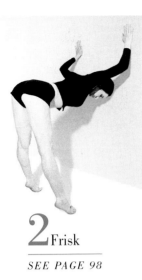

2 Frisk

SEE PAGE 98

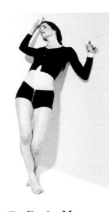

3 Brain Massage Turn

SEE PAGE 100

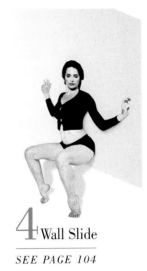

4 Wall Slide

SEE PAGE 104

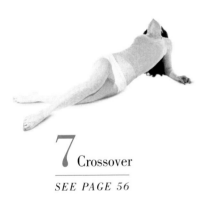

7 Crossover

SEE PAGE 56

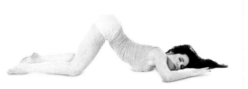

8 Cat Pounce

SEE PAGE 62

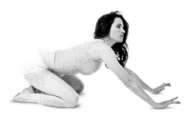

9 Cat Pounce Hip Circles

SEE PAGE 62

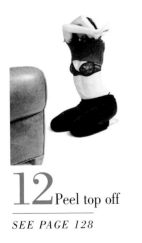

12 Peel top off

SEE PAGE 128

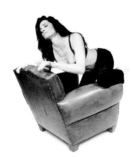

13 Lap Dance

SEE PAGE 142

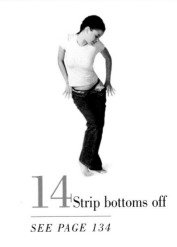

14 Strip bottoms off

SEE PAGE 134

the new guy strip

Got a new guy in your life? Pique his interest by revealing just a bit of skin (but take it slow and don't give away the whole show . . . yet).

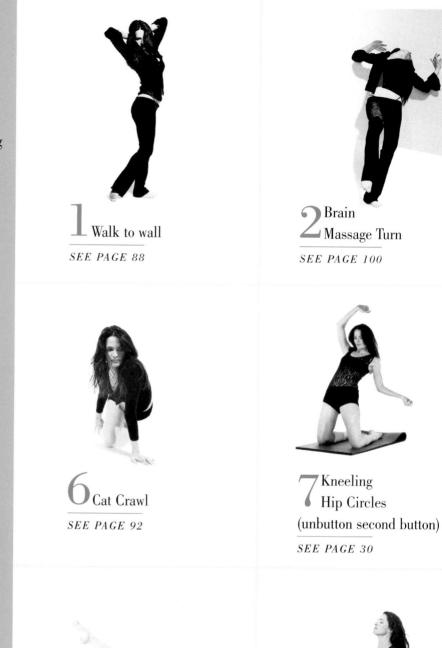

1 Walk to wall

SEE PAGE 88

2 Brain Massage Turn

SEE PAGE 100

6 Cat Crawl

SEE PAGE 92

7 Kneeling Hip Circles (unbutton second button)

SEE PAGE 30

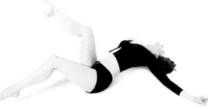

11 Prancing Goddess

SEE PAGE 84

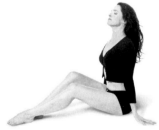

12 Goddess Rising

SEE PAGE 86

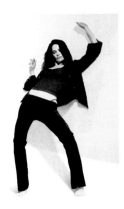

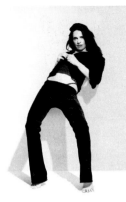

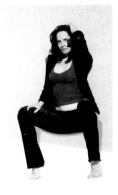

3 Wall Hip Circles

SEE PAGE 102

4 Unbutton first button

SEE PAGE 126

5 Wall Slide down

SEE PAGE 104

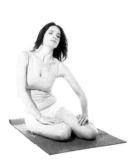

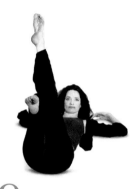

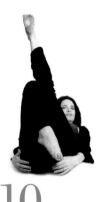

8 Mermaid (onto back)

SEE PAGE 74

9 Peel Up

SEE PAGE 44

10 Flirt

SEE PAGE 50

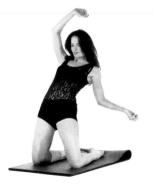

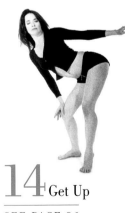

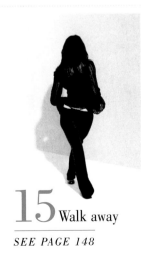

13 Kneeling Hip Circles (unbutton third button)

SEE PAGE 30

14 Get Up

SEE PAGE 96

15 Walk away

SEE PAGE 148

special valentine's day strip

Sexier than heart panties, smokier than a box of cigars, more powerful than Cupid's arrow, the Valentine's Day Strip is the quickest way to your man's heart.

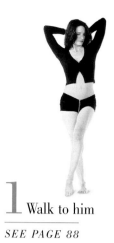

1 Walk to him

SEE PAGE 88

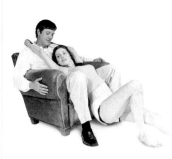

2 Lap Dance with Back Body Slide dismount

SEE PAGE 142

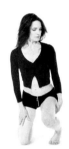

6 Get Up

SEE PAGE 96

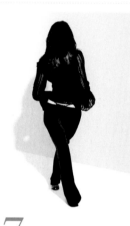

7 Walk to wall

SEE PAGE 148

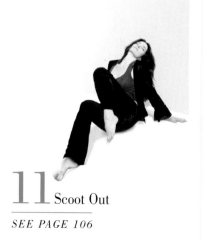

11 Scoot Out

SEE PAGE 106

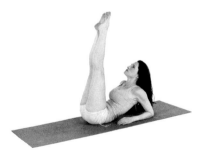

12 Peel Up

SEE PAGE 44

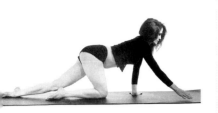

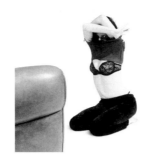

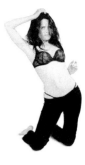

3 Cat Crawl
away

SEE PAGE 92

4 Peel top off

SEE PAGE 128

5 Kneeling Hip
Circles

SEE PAGE 30

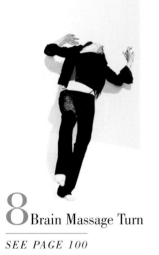

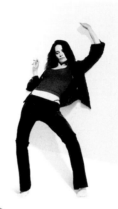

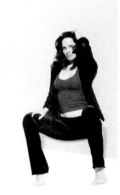

8 Brain Massage Turn

SEE PAGE 100

9 Wall Hip Circles

SEE PAGE 102

10 Wall Slide

SEE PAGE 104

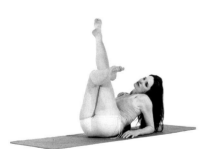

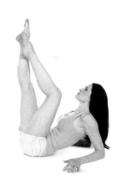

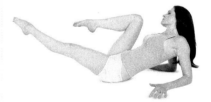

13 Flirt

SEE PAGE 50

14 Fiddler

SEE PAGE 46

15 Prance

SEE PAGE 48

special valentine's day strip (continued)

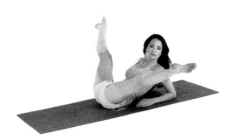

16 Leg Splay
SEE PAGE 52

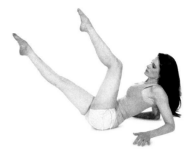

17 Prance
SEE PAGE 48

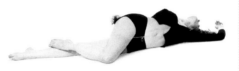

21 Crossover
SEE PAGE 56

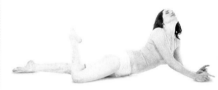

22 Belly Roll
SEE PAGE 61

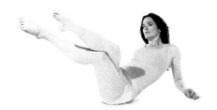

26 Peel Up
SEE PAGE 44

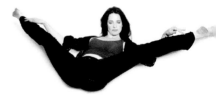

27 Leg Splay
SEE PAGE 52

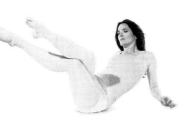

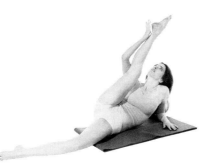

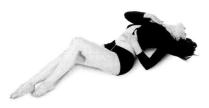

18 Crossover

SEE PAGE 56

19 Side Leg Peel

SEE PAGE 58

20 Writhing Goddess

SEE PAGE 82

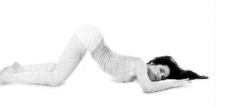

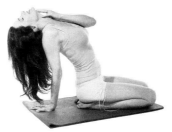

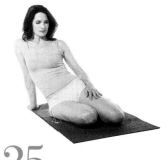

23 Cat Pounce

SEE PAGE 62

24 Picasso Arch

SEE PAGE 64

25 Mermaid

SEE PAGE 74

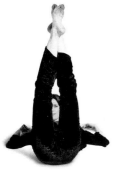

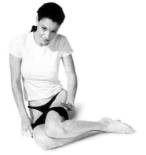

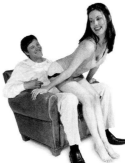

28 Fiddler

SEE PAGE 46

29 Mermaid (pull bottoms off)

SEE PAGE 74

30 Lap Dance (you should be in underwear)

SEE PAGE 142

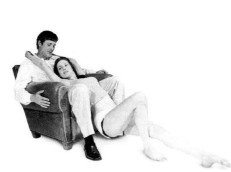

31 Back Body Slide

SEE PAGE 143

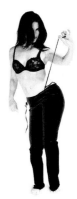

32 Standing Hip Circles (tug at G-string)

SEE PAGE 32

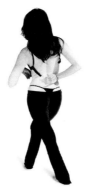

33 Walk away as you unsnap your bra

SEE PAGE 136

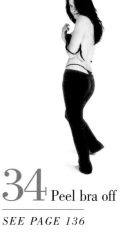

34 Peel bra off

SEE PAGE 136

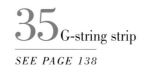

35 G-string strip

SEE PAGE 138

36

The rest is history!

BONUS...Pick your Stripper Name

Over the years, exotic dancers have created stripper names for themselves—Blaze Starr, Tempest Storm, Lily St. Cyr, to name a few. Even today you can be pretty sure that the strip dancers' names are aliases. They say they do it to protect their identities, but then why not just use Jane or Sue? I think the names strippers pick are fun, colorful descriptions of their erotic alter egos. Below are some of the names I've heard in the clubs. Have some fun: take two names and put them together. For your first name, choose one from list A that describes your erotic creature; for your second name, choose one from list B that describes her sensual tastes or pleasures.

A

TOMBOY: *Frankie, Alex, Charlie, Joey, Danny, Devon, Rocky, Spike*

GOLD DIGGER: *Gold or Goldie, Silver, Diamond, Platinum, Emerald, Ruby, Opal, Porsche, Mercedes, Lexus, Fendi, Chanel, Sterling, Mink, Tiffany, Crystal, Sparkle, Jewel, Jade*

NATURAL WONDERS: *Lake, Everest, River, Amazon, Mirage, Oasis*

EARTHY: *Dune/Duney, Ivy, Eartha, Willow, Meadow, Woodstock*

FRANCOPHILE: *Colette, Gigi, Coco, Lulu, Lola, Lolita, Fifi, Simone*

ROYAL: *Queen, Duchess, Princess, Lady*

BAD-ASS: *Sin, Jezebel, Blaze, Delilah, Cleopatra/Cleo, Xena, Eve, Lilith, Poison Ivy*

ALL OVER THE MAP: *China, India, Europa, Argentina, Dakota, Montana, Carolina, Houston, Dallas, Paris, Sahara, Russia, Asia, Jamaica, Havana, Riviera, Arizona, Cheyenne, Phoenix*

B

INTOXICATING: *Bourbon, Tequila, Brandy, Martini, Champagne, Crystal, Merlot, Chardonnay*

CELESTIAL/ATMOSPHERIC: *Sky/Skye, Cloudy, Misty, Storm, Rain, Sunny, Starlight/Star, Luna, Venus, Snowy, Icy, Dusty, Tempest, Mercury*

WILD: *Lynx, Cobra, Mink, Cheetah, Ibex, Gazelle, Puma, Jaguar, Tiger, Cougar, Falcon*

FLOWER CHILD: *Violet, Daisy, Begonia, Rose, Jasmine, Heather, Poppy, Holly, Deflora*

SPICE GIRL: *Ginger, Pepper, Anise, Cayenne, Cardamom*

YUMMY: *Apple, Cherry, Strawberry, Peaches, Sugar, Cookie, Candy, Honey*

SWEET: *Barbie, Bunny, Angel, Kitten, Bambi, Birdie, Baby/Babydoll, Betty, Sweet*

SEASONAL/TIMELY: *Summer, Autumn, Winter, June, May, April, December, Spring, Tuesday*

TOUCHABLE: *Velvet, Satin, Lacy, Silk, Cashmere, Angora, Velour*

COLORFUL: *Ruby, Azure, Silver, Chartreuse, Neon, Amber, Ebony, Pink, Scarlet, Turquoise*

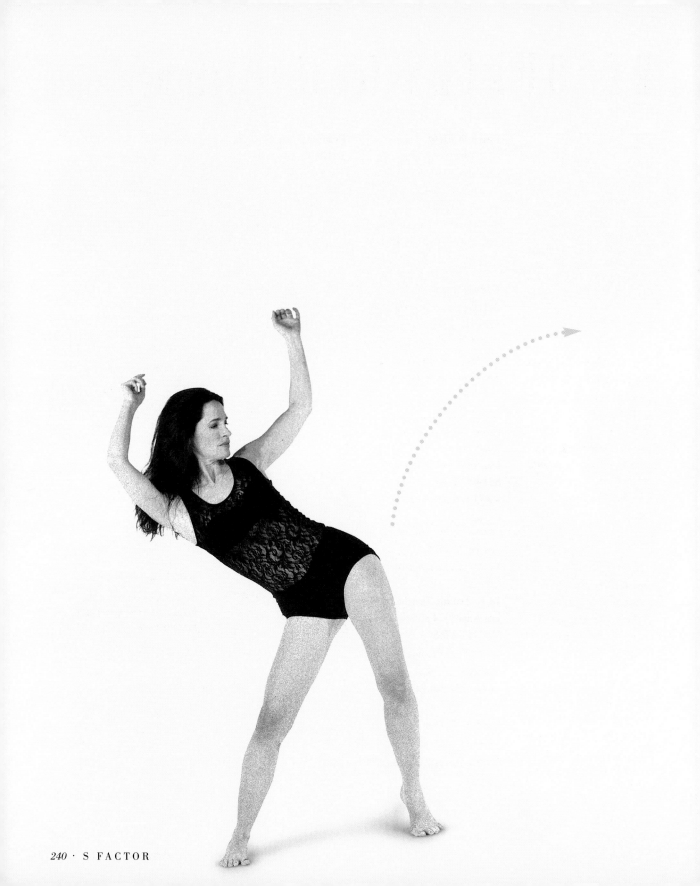

RESOURCES for the Stripper

THE S FACTOR

Los Angeles, California
323-965-9685
www.sfactor.com
e-mail: info@sfactor.com

*In addition to offering
S Factor classes, the online
store offers poles, T-shirts,
G-strings, videos, and other
fun stuff.*

CLOTHING & ACCESSORIES

Frederick's of Hollywood
800-323-9525
www.fredericks.com
*see Web site for a store
location near you.*

*Lingerie, high heels, wigs,
costumes, and sexy clothing*

Forplay Catalog
www.forplaycatalog.com
*Clothing, dancewear,
and shoes*

Sensual Looks
www.sensuallooks.com
*Full stripper costumes,
including French maid,
cowgirl, military, and
baby doll*

The Stripper Zone
www.stripperzone.com
e-mail: info@stripperzone.com
*Comprehensive site includes
accessories, clothing, lingerie,
and shoes*

Patricia Field
New York, New York
212-966-4066
www.patriciafield.com
*The Sex and the City stylist
carries vinyl hot pants, wigs,
body glitter, lingerie, and
boas.*

Roma Bikini
Los Angeles, California
323-957-1988
e-mail: romabikini@aol.com
*Specializes in teeny-weeny
bikinis and sexy dancer
clothing*

SHOES

Tony Shoes, Inc.
Los Angeles, California
323-467-5604
www.tonyshoesinc.com
e-mail:
tonyshoes@tonyshoesinc.com
*6- and 8-inch heels in a
variety of styles and colors*

Lady Studio Exotic Shoes
Los Angeles, California
323-461-1765
www.ladystudioshoes.com
*6- and 8-inch heels in a
variety of styles and colors*

Sensual Looks
www.sensuallooks.com
Boots, stilettos, platforms

Pennangalan Dreams
15 Gloucester Avenue
Slough, SL1 #AW
United Kingdom
+44 (0) 1753-678076
www.pennangalan.co.uk
Mostly boots

SEXY LINGERIE

Biatta
www.biatta.com
Available at Bloomingdale's
and Macy's

On Gossamer
www.ongossamer.com
*See Web site for a store
location near you.*

Victoria's Secret
www.victoriassecret.com
*See Web site for a store
location near you.*

Agent Provocateur
New York, New York
www.agentprovocateur.com

La Perla
www.laperla.com

Undiemoon
www.undiemoon.com
e-mail:
undies@undiemoon.com

Cosabella
www.cosabella.com

Only Hearts
www.onlyhearts.com

DANCING POLES

The S Factor
1-866-4THESFACTOR
www.sfactor.com
e-mail: info@sfactor.com

Kegworks
www.kegworks.com
*Under "Commercial
Equipment," you'll
find dancer poles.*

The Stripper Zone
www.stripperzone.com
e-mail: info@stripperzone.com
A variety of poles

Dry Hands
1-888-258-4696
www.dryhands.com
*A nonsticky solution that
helps keep your hands dry
for pole work*